"When given the choice between being right or being kind, choose kind"

R J PALACIO, WONDER

Afterwards - The Postpartum Spectacle
Copyright © 2021 by Tori Bowman Johnson

———————————

Written by Tori Bowman Johnson
www.afterwardspostpartum.com.au | @afterwards.postpartum
tori@jandvco.com

Illustrated by Catherine Malady

Printed by Discus on Demand | HP7600 Indigo press
www.discusondemand.com.au

In honour of my good friend Elyse Knowles who lives to protect nature, this book is printed using recycled paper material.

Designed by Goya Studio
www.goyastudio.com.au | @goya_studio

ISBN: 978-0-6452631-0-7

AFTER-WARDS

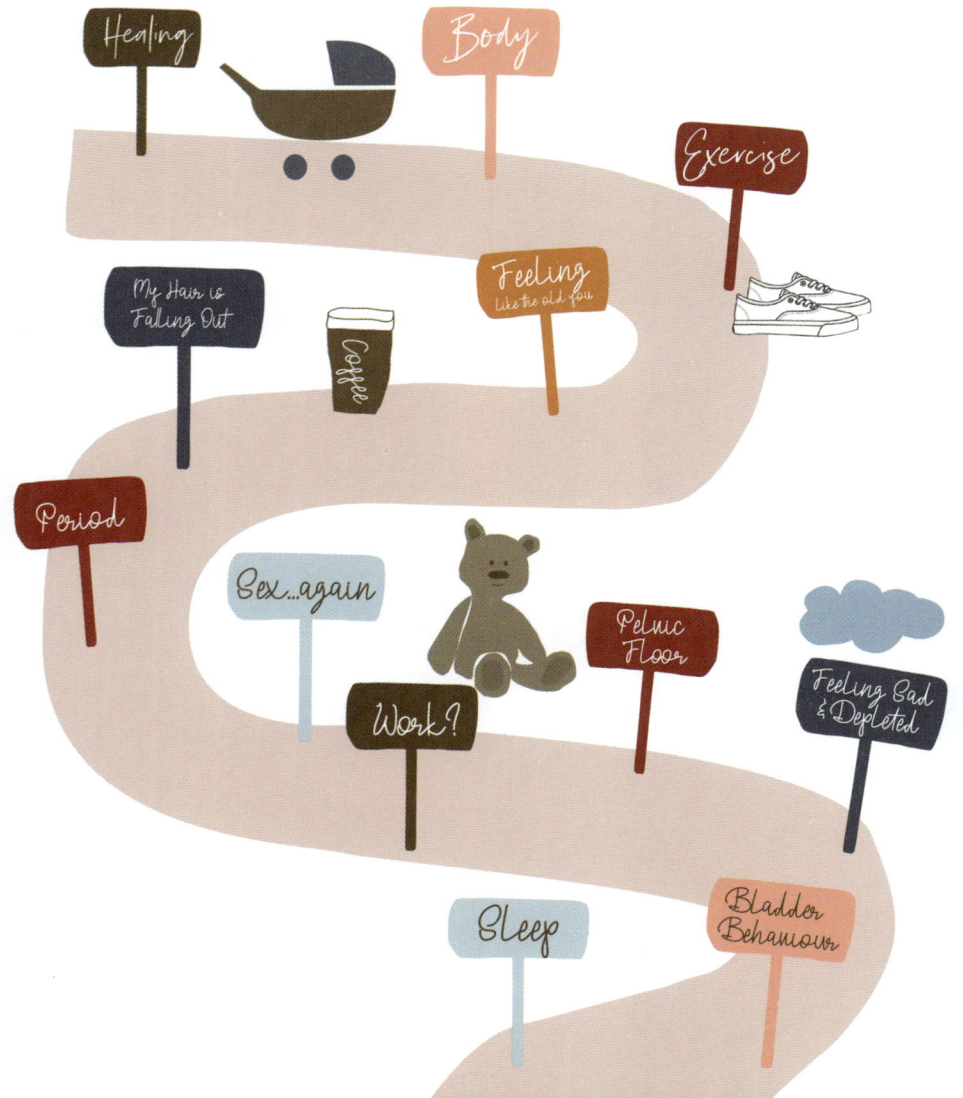

TO MY LITTLE MAN HAMISH.

FOR REMINDING ME THAT LITTLE NEVER MEANS LESS. LITTLE IS GENEROUS AS IT'S LIFE'S LITTLE THINGS THAT PROVIDE GREATER SPACES FOR BIG LOVE TO EXIST.

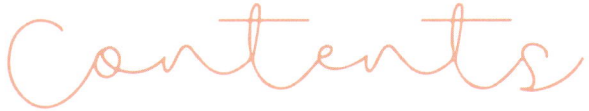

FOREWORD	**P09**
INTRODUCTION	**P13**
CHAPTER 1 / THE BODY	**P27**
CHAPTER 2 / THE PELVIC FLOOR	**P53**
CHAPTER 3 / BOOBS	**P61**
CHAPTER 4 / POO. PADS & PIDDLES	**P79**
CHAPTER 5 / SEX	**P95**
CHAPTER 6 / POSTPARTUM & THE BIG C	**P111**
CHAPTER 7 / VANITY	**P121**
CHAPTER 8 / MR. GUILT	**P133**
CHAPTER 9 / BOREDOM	**P149**
CHAPTER 10 / HEALING	**P159**
CHAPTER 11 / WHEN IT'S NOT POSTNATAL DEPRESSION	**P171**
THANK YOU	**P177**

FOREWORD

On Christmas Day 1989, the year after my brother was born & the year before I came along, my Mum gave her Dad (my Poppy), a book. The Complete Tales of Beatrix Potter. It was an original & authorised edition and Mum had handwritten Pop's name under the words, This Book Belongs To.

30 years on in 2019, my Nan gifted me this book when I was pregnant with my son. Just like Poppy had read it to me, I can now share these sweetly nostalgic stories with my Hamish. There is something warm & significant about books when they're shared through generations. Like vintage jewels, the printed words and torn pages prevail the novelties of newness.

I invite you to leave your mark below, and go on to pass Afterwards down to your own daughter or someone else close. In no way will the charming stories of Beatrix Potter compare to the themes of this book … however like other tales, Afterwards may punctuate a moment in time. A moment you felt vulnerable and wonderful… so sleepy while hovering in a hyper haze. A moment where day was night, and night was day. A moment that words may never mature enough to articulate the way it feels to become a mother for the first time.

Yes it's messy and yes it is intense. Even though, the postpartum existence is a collection of raw moments that should bring women together. No matter the time, no matter the day, no matter the year.

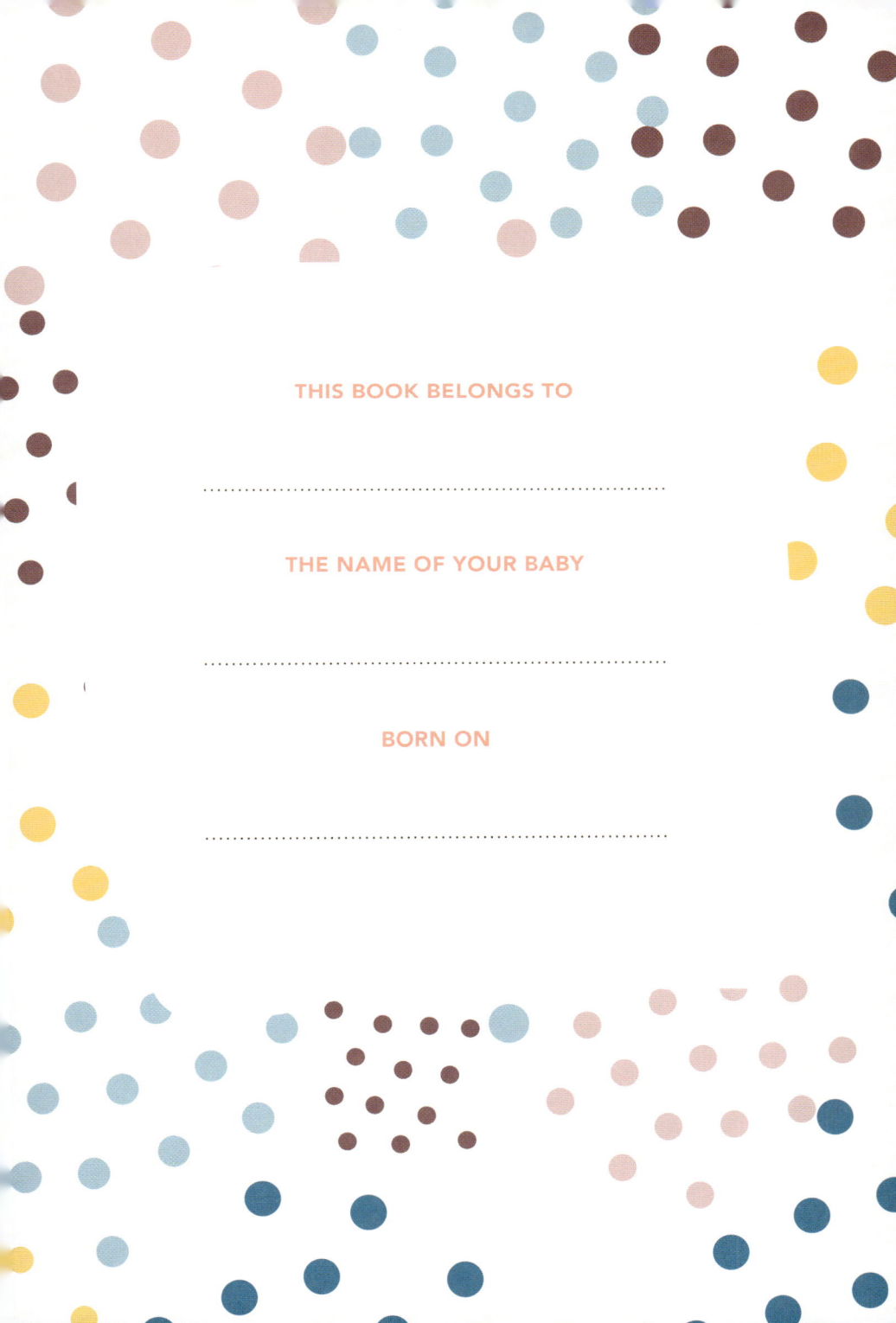

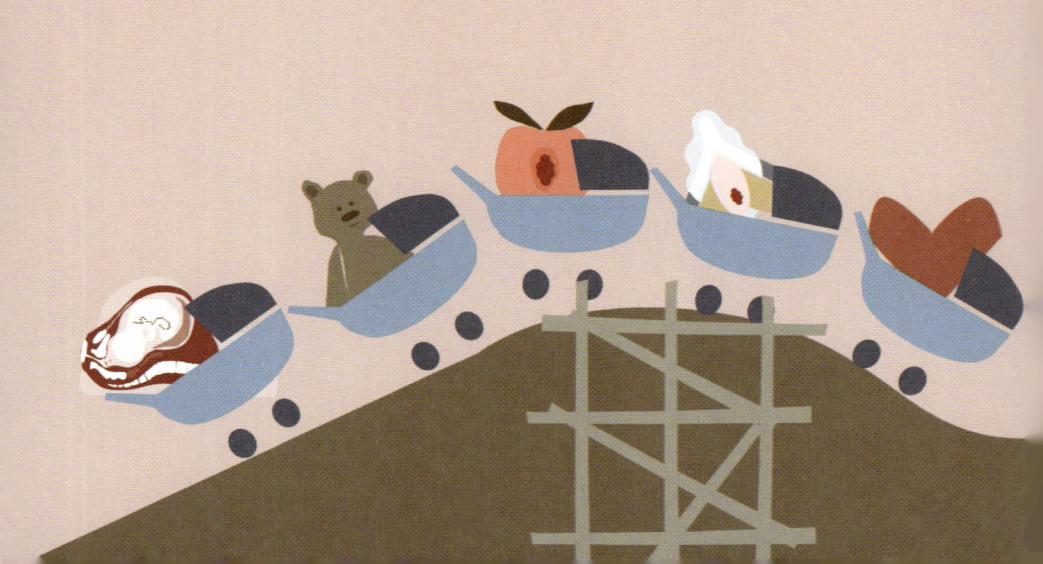

Introduction

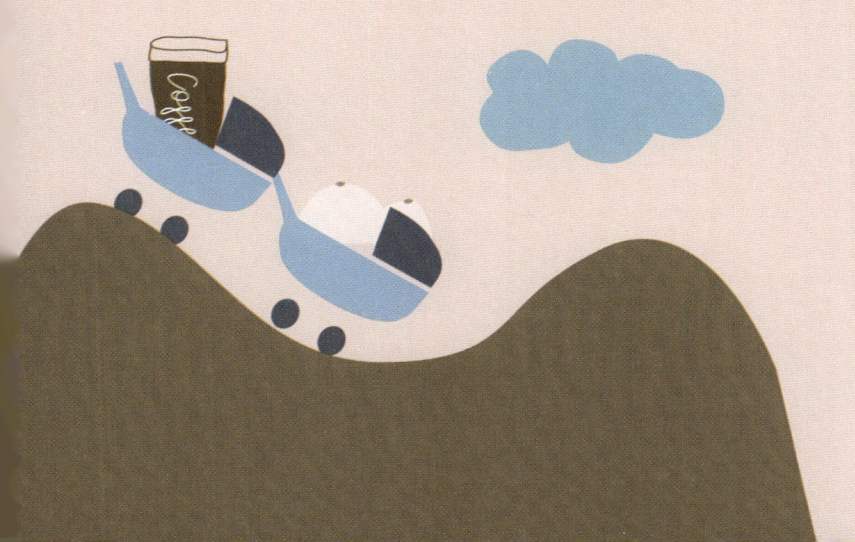

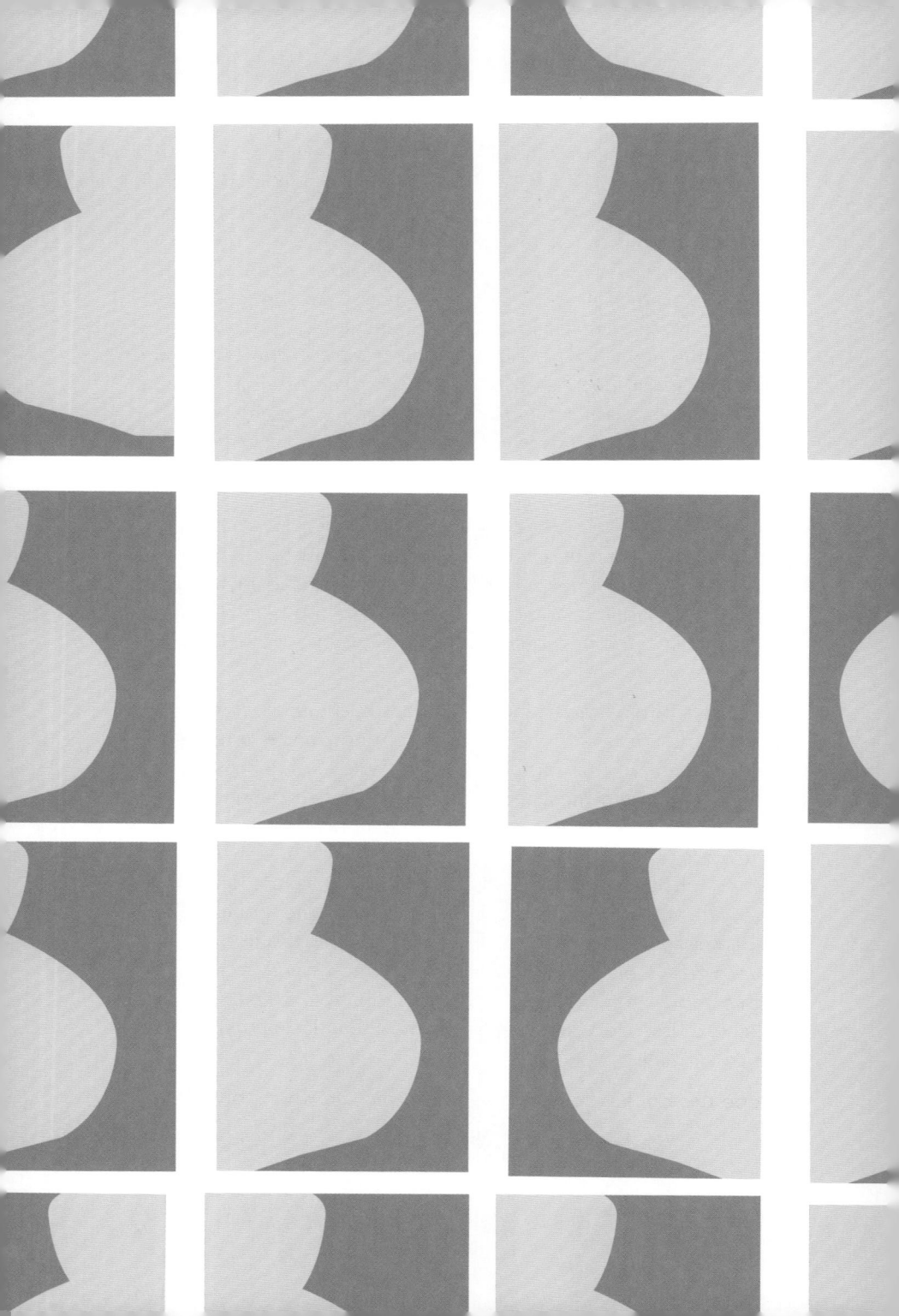

Having a baby for the first time is a little like moving to a foreign country & sharing a hostel dorm with someone you've never met before. You both speak very different languages and therefore communication is tricky. You've come from different countries so your sleep patterns take a while to sync up … and the jet lag you're both dealing with is relentless and slow to ease. Your new roommate is small & petite but their snoring and grunting through the night is alarming. You almost want to wake them and ask if they're OK because you are truly shocked by what you hear. Their bathroom habits could use some work … and their table manners are far & few between but they're traveling with you every day and co-creating some beautiful adventures. Together you laugh often and rediscover the best part of a friendship. The unpredictability and spontaneous nature of your days both feed your adrenaline and unravel a new kind of exhaustion. This trip you're on … this wild experience you share is unlike anything you could have imagined. You feel lucky to have met them & grateful to know them. You now believe in soulmates as you have found your own.

I hope this book offers some laughs for new Mums & some insights and answers to the things that bring wonder or worry. Birth is beautiful, as is raising a baby but the experience also brings a LOT of newness into the life of a woman…especially in terms of her body. There are so many things that could lead to shyness or embarrassment as the control you once had over your body is now in the past. New Mums have enough to deal with when they're in the thick of newborn life. Feelings of embarrassment or loneliness need to be eradicated from all households where a new Mum with a newborn lives, so the aim of this book is to lay everything out on the table & keep any and all fears at bay. Poo, sex, bladder control, hair loss, confusion. We cover it all!

I hope this book is something you can pick up when you're

feeling curious but you're too tired to get caught up in a sea of Google searches. I hope it's something you pass onto a friend when she needs a hint of support or just a good laugh. I truly hope your experience as a new Mumma is everything you hoped it would be. And if it's not, go easy on yourself. A wonderful rhythm will find you, a wave of confidence will wash over you and when you least expect it, your own style of mothering will become effortlessly intuitive (even if it looks chaotic to everyone around you). Avoid rushing to get there though ...

Your pace, your baby, your story.

Here we go!

...

It might be because I didn't listen too closely during human biology (I can't even remember if I took the elective to be honest), however, I was fairly oblivious to all matters regarding the female anatomy until after my son was born. Sure I knew the main bits & bobs ... head, shoulders, knees & toes ... eyes and ears and mouth and nose ... but the nitty-gritty? No clue.

The reproductive system? Zilch!

When it came to menstruation, I knew that my period came once a month and if my boobs hurt or if my mood was short & shitty, I could simply file it away under the category; PMS. I knew that I'd need to use contraception until I was ready to try for a baby with my partner and I was pretty sure that when my period was late there was a good chance a baby was on its merry way. And about 9 months ago, he was.

What did I know from the point of falling pregnant? Not a lot. I knew that A) I'd grow a belly, B) I'd need a bigger bra, and C); I'd have funny food cravings and I would need to pee at all times.

So after weeing on the stick and reading those celebrated words, "3-4 weeks pregnant", the next 40weeks were all about growing and cherishing the little person who was blissfully housed in my body.

And then…. come week 40+1, that little person (we now call him Hamish), came out and holy moly did the experience blow my mind. Birth is ex-f**ing-treme. Oh my good gosh is it ever. In the weeks & months that followed, I became fueled by an imploding curiosity about my body and the mix of incredible, natural & let's be honest … traumatising series of events it had just endured.

I use the word traumatising lightly, sure there were traumatic moments during my son's birth. It was long, painful & not exactly what you'd call "smooth sailing." Adding to this, straight after his birth I fell into a state of sheer shock & confusion (more on that later), however in the grand scheme of things it was a very successful delivery and I can happily say my experience was nothing short of phenomenal. The midwives and doctors present were fantastic & lay a very healthy little boy on my chest at 4.44am on the 31st of December 2019.

I'd love to tell you all that I birthed comfortably within a few blissful hours layered in hypnobirthing calmness, essential oils & positive affirmations … but this wasn't my story…and I'm sure that while it could very much be your next birthing story, it probably wasn't your experience this time around either.

My story included a few super cute characters such as Ian the Induction featuring Betty the Balloon, Eddie the Epidural (… and his very capable understudy Edwina since Eddie suffered a bad case of stage fright), Frank the Forceps, Emma the Episiotomy, Henry the Hemorrhage and Bob … the short term but deeply terrifying Black Hole of "I Am Broken, Someone Help Me Please." Bob especially, was a real little show stopper to who I'd have to award rave reviews. He stopped me in my tracks. His performance made me cry, shake with terror, and beg the midwife to turn the volume right down as the post-birth dip was simply too much to bear.

But even though my story sounds a little glum & Bob sounds like the villain who would haunt you in your dreams, it was a great birth and Bob pissed right off soon after.

I was in great medical hands. I had a healthy baby boy & my darling partner by my side. My mind & body returned to a healthy state and I feel grateful and very fortunate.

So if you were to ask me, "Was your birth traumatic?", I'd happily say no.

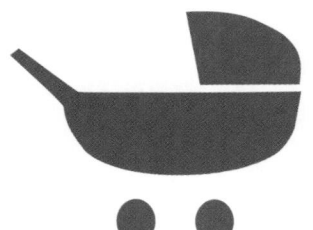

But.

If you asked my vagina? If you asked ANY woman's vagina or the abdomen of a woman who underwent a C-Section, "Was your birth traumatic?" I think they would reply with ease "What The F*** Do You Think?"

They'd have the right to reply to this question with explosive passion and a profanity or twenty. They have been poked with tools and flooded with hormones. They've been stretched, cut & torn. They've been bruised, stitched, iced, and exhausted in all meanings of the word.

I know this sounds gruesome but folks, this is the miracle of life.

I now sit here writing this book 9 months after birthing my son & while I of course remember the pain, the fluorescent lighting, the machine beeps, the fear of the unknown, and the many clinical elements. I remember the shock my mind collapsed into & the hunger... the desperate need to eat after he was delivered. Sure, I remember my first shower (which can only be described as something you'd see in an R18+ Sci-Fi film) and it'll be hard to ever forget the tears I shed when I bought my baby home and felt a deep sense of sadness. As unusual as it sounds I was so upset that he wasn't physically connected to me, anymore. While he was in my arms, I mourned the fact he was no longer in my belly.

I remember it all.

But would I do it all over again?

YES!!

After what I've just written about birth, my excitement sounds completely messed up ... right? Truly, what kind of sicko voluntarily signs up for that sequence of events twice. Are women a little coo-coo? No such luck. Women are very brave, resilient, capable & seriously driven. Women hold a body that creates new life.

Anyway, before I start singing Aretha Franklin & quoting Gloria Steinman, I'll explain what this book is about and why I'm writing it now, 9months after having my baby boy Hamish.

Think back to the start of this chapter where I touched on my lack of human biology knowledge. It's, for this reason, I felt the urge to write this book. I feel that all women, including myself, owe it to their bodies to really get to know them inside & out. With knowledge comes power & trust. Two things you need when you birth a baby & nurse your body back to health.

As I said, my son, Hamish is now 9 months old, meaning he's been earth side for as long as he was cocooned inside of my body. Only now, however, am I really grasping onto what actually happened to my body during pregnancy, labour & what is continuing to happen to my body all these months later.

Within the first few weeks following your birth when you're told to rest & recover until your 6 week check-up, you count down the minutes with tremendous anticipation. You read books such as The First Six Weeks by Midwife Cath as if it's the holy bible & you hold onto such weighted hope that come your 6 week check-up, your GP will hand you a framed certificate that reads, "YOU PASSED! You are ALL fixed up & back to your pre-baby self! High Five!"

Ok, so spoiler alert for those reading who are expecting. The recovery process is not quite refined to 6 weeks. It's sort of like when people refer to "24/7 sickness", during pregnancy as "morning sickness." In other words, in many cases, it is a gross exaggeration.

Usually, 6 weeks is a drop in the ocean. Before you stress though, unclench your tensed body as this isn't such a bad thing. Recovering from birth doesn't have to translate to pain, tears, and chronic angst. Absolutely not. It just means that your body needs more time (in some cases, a lot more time) to recoup from what was an undeniably traumatic experience.

Over the last 9 months, I've become more curious and more amazed by how clever & intuitive our bodies are. I've also become a lot kinder to my body. That old cliché saying, "listen to your body," has taken on a whole new meaning. It birthed a human after all. A human! The least I can do is let it sleep when it needs to sleep & feed it a few extra treats when it asks for "more please".

More importantly, however, since expanding my human biology knowledge and self-awareness, I can now better conceptualise that there is both a physical & mental side of birth and the marriage between the two is intuitively connected. While we may feel a certain way, we need to avoid assuming our bodies will always agree on a physical level.

Here's a quick example to illustrate the point I'm getting at. About 8 weeks after giving birth, I felt full of energy and so excited to get back to an exercise class. My body looked normal-ish on the outside, my stitches had healed & my boobs were controllable as long as I wore nipple pads and a very supportive sports bra. So off I went to F45.

I went a littleeee red in the face when after just one light jump lunge, I thought to myself, "Did I just wee? Surely not!" Well as it tuned out, yes I did. I wet my pants. Awesome.

Since investigating why this happened and why I lacked the self-control I assumed I had, I now get it. I now understand why my body didn't send me the warning sign, "Pee Coming, Find Toilet." The reason? My body didn't know my bladder was about to prank us either. The delightful surprise splash of wee was due to a weak & very tired pelvic floor. Nothing was broken but my body was simply not ready for any kind of nonessential impact. It was still healing & it did not appreciate me bouncing around like an excitable toddler.

After this experience I didn't stop going to the gym, I just made alterations to my workout (many) & specified what I could and couldn't do *yet*. I stress the word *yet* as it's important to note that returning to the activities you enjoyed pre-baby is not

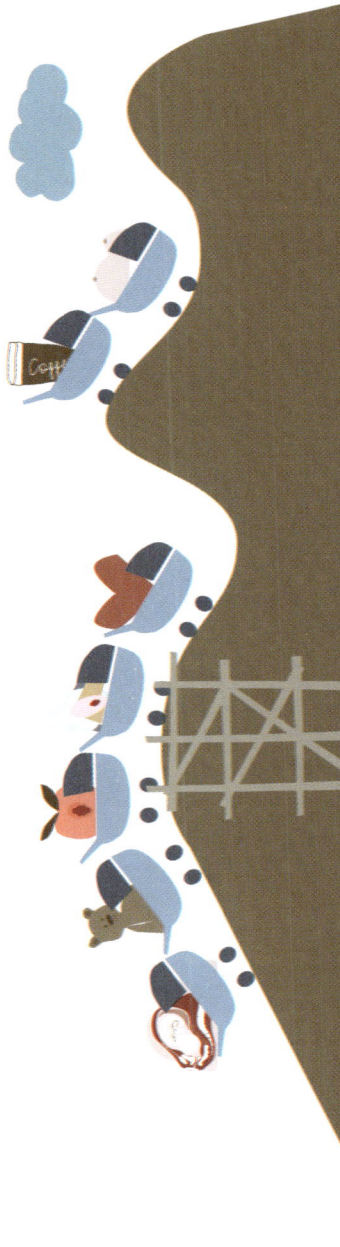

impossible, but it's also not a race. It's a process. And every new Mum's process is different, so throw out any plans you had to compare yourself to the Mum next door.

Since diving into my curious bodily queries & learning more about the body versus the mind, I can now compartmentalise what my body endured over the 9 months of pregnancy & I can wrap my head around what has happened over the 9 months since. Having an improved self-awareness has had quite a substantial impact on my mindset & dare I say, the speed of my recovery. It feels a little like having a birds-eye view of the road ahead and using this view to foresee & avoid as many roadblocks or detours as possible.

So now when I'm riddled with worry or stressing over thoughts such as Is my body abnormal? Am I broken? Will I ever feel the same? I'm able to rationally process the emotional thought & calmly tell myself ... Calm the hell down lady! You just pushed a baby out of your body so put the brakes on the star jumps, grab some toast and watch another episode of Grey's Anatomy.

With some basic knowledge, rest, patience, and professional guidance, women can dramatically help their physical selves bounce back beautifully. With confidence, you can create a new version of normal for yourself and feel really great about it. But the 6 week postpartum time frame that seems to be drilled into our expectations post-birth? It's a cruel tease so best to turn the page on that one.

6 weeks might cover the time needed to allow your stitches to dissolve, your uterus to retract, your boobs to soften and your milk to regulate. 6 weeks might cover the time needed for your bleeding to stop, your mind to reason with the thought of having sex again, your night sweats to dry out and your perineum to heal.

But ...

Weeks 7, 8, 9, 10, 20, 30, 40 ...., and so forth? The weeks proceeding will continue to uncover & introduce new challenges, aches, and weakened muscles that once boasted strength. And guess what? That is OK! It's perfectly NORMAL and it's TO BE EXPECTED. While I bet you're not stoked about it, you're also not alone. You're human.

The other thing you're not alone in? Worrying about the nitty-gritty bits and bobs post-birth. The stuff you think shouldn't matter because it's unrelated to the health of your baby. But this "stuff" shouldn't be discounted as it's the stuff that matters to you.

New Mums seem to be missing too much information regarding subjects that go hand-in-hand with flushed cheeks & embarrassment for many. And embarrassment can manifest into bigger issues if you let it compromise your recovery. For this reason, the soul of this book is to help women eradicate their embarrassment by getting right into a bunch of subjects that you may subconsciously pair with stigma, shame or awkwardness.

What kind of subjects am I referring to? Things like the ability to ask your GP or even a close friend/fellow Mum about your lost sex drive. The appearance of your vagina or your regularity. Fear around returning to the beautician due to thoughts such as, "What if it's carnage down there?" (Another spoiler alert; Your vagina heals. It is not carnage.)

Subjects such as asking your partner to bring you an extra towel so you can wipe up the bathroom floor as you've wet yourself… again. How to stay clean and hygienic with stitches in all kinds of odd areas. The list is endless!

You feel so undignified after having a baby in so many ways. You wake to milk and sweat sodden sheets, you stuff your underwear with pads larger than your newborn's nappies and icepacks & you sit alone in the dark at 2am thinking to yourself … I am sore, I am tired and I am frustrated. I have lost all control over my body, my time, myself.

I sincerely empathise with any woman feeling these things as it can feel brutal. It can feel joyless and lonely and terrifyingly suffocating as you think to yourself, I don't recognise my own life anymore.

So let's make it easier for ourselves, for our friends, our sisters, our daughters, our colleagues. Let's just lay the gory, the unpleasant & the distressing questions about everything "icky" on the table and get right to the point so new Mums can quit feeling alone and undesirable & instead reassure themselves that they're OK.

Quick Warning: The aim of this book is not to provide medical guidance or parental advice. I'm not a psychologist, a physio, a midwife … nor am I a mother of multiple children with years & years of child-rearing experience. I'm simply a new Mum with a whole lot of questions and endless curiosity about the body that grew my baby.

With this in mind, the aim of this book is to sharpen the familiarity you share with your own body. With some fabulous professionals in the women's health space, this book should allow you to holistically understand what your body is doing (or trying to do) when recovering from birth. The book will cover some tips & tricks, it'll shed light on grim areas (i.e. doing your first poo after birth) and it will make you smile. Because being a Mum is all kinds of fun. Let's be honest.

So how are we going to do all of this? Easy! Using simple diagrams, cute pictures & laymen's terms! Why? Because this book all started back when I was far too embarrassed to ask my GP;

"Exactly what the hell is going on? A few months ago I bathed my big belly in delicious essential oils, nesting in the most poetic of ways. Now I'm icing an area you tell me is called my perineum & 6 weeks later I can't work out if it's my vagina or my butt."

So off we go. Let's explore this colossal, chaotic existence people like to call, postpartum life!

WAIT! Before we get any further into this book, let's quickly cover one very important topic first. Contraception! I'm sure there are many first time Mums who would love to grow a big & bustling brood of children, which is amazing! Prior to diving back into the baby pool again however, it might be worth letting your body heal first.

For more on this topic our midwife extraordinaire, Sophie Outhwaite chimes in to share a few other factors to be wary of ...

Why do all the midwives, doctors, GP's, maternal health nurses etc all seem to obsess over contraception, just days (or even hours!) after a woman gives birth?

Unplanned pregnancies! There seems to be a vicious rumour floating around that women cannot conceive while breastfeeding. Women can and do fall pregnant immediately after birth. Even if you've not yet menstruated, you may ovulate and therefore may conceive. Compounding this fact, is research suggesting short interpregnancy intervals have been associated with adverse perinatal outcomes such as an increased risk of preterm birth, low birth weights and small for gestational age babies*.

*Conde-Agudelo A, Rosas-Bermúdez A, Kafury-Goeta AC. Birth spacing and risk of adverse perinatal outcomes: a meta-analysis. JAMA. 2006 Apr 19;295(15):1809-23. doi: 10.1001/jama.295.15.1809. PMID: 16622143.

Ok! So now that we have covered that, let's move on. If you want to read about contraceptive methods, whether it's the pill, the mini pill, an IUD (i.e. the Mirena®), the NuvaRing®, condoms etc - it's best to speak openly (and quickly), with your GP.

CHAPTER 1
the body

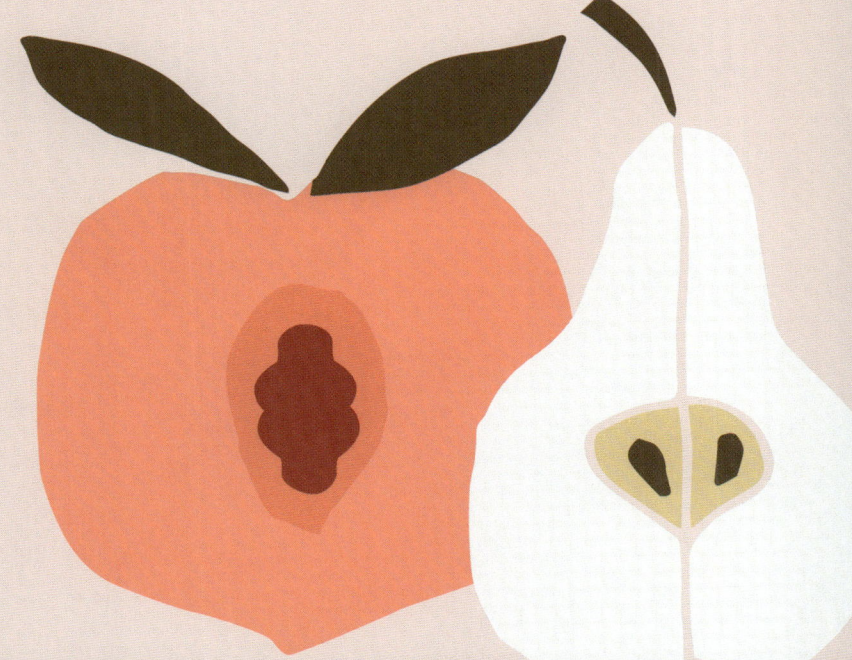

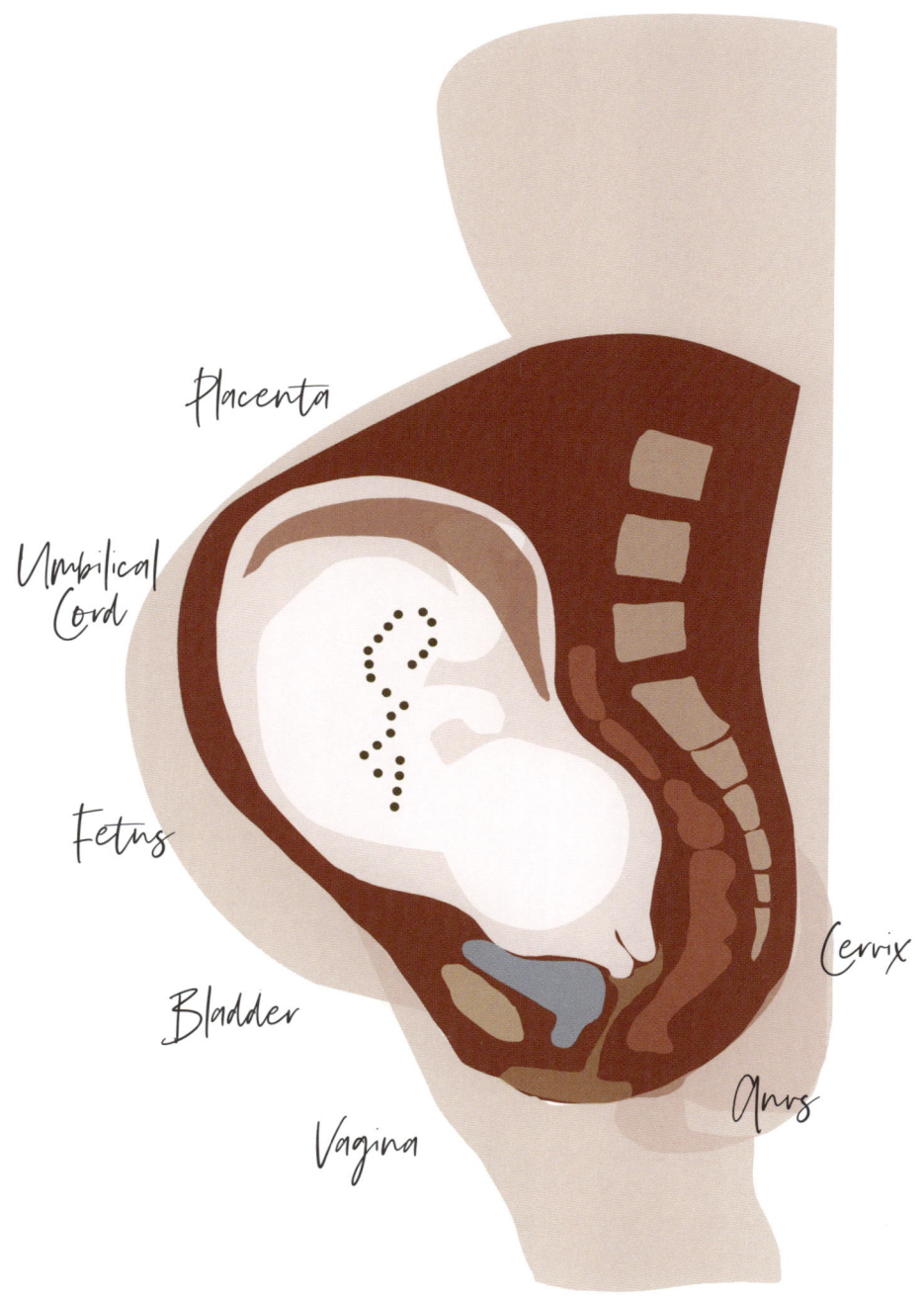

Let's start up the top. Well actually, let's start south of the boob region as we've dedicated them their very own chapter in the coming pages (they deserve the extra cred!).

To kick things off… the belly! The place we carry the baby! Well, sort of. We don't actually carry babies in our bellies like we imagined we did as kids. Close but not quite. We carry babies in;

THE UTERUS

So what is & where is the uterus? In the simplest of explanations, the uterus sits above your vagina. As your baby grows bigger and bigger, a woman's uterus will expand into the stomach area causing their belly to grow simultaneously… hence the bump. This may be obvious to some, however not to all.

If you feel an influx of hideous cramps after having your baby (similar, however potentially more chronic than menstrual cramps), these pains may be related to the contraction of your uterus, especially if you are breastfeeding. As the uterus works hard to shrink back to it's pre-baby size, this process involves a compression of the blood vessels which in turn controls the intensity of postpartum bleeding. It's likely these cramps will last a period of days or weeks but do be wary as they can be quite sharp & severe. Rumor has it they can be worse for your 2nd or 3rd baby. Apologies for being the bearer of bad news! If you are worried about the pain and need help managing it, as always the best thing to do is give your midwife or your GP a bell. If the pain is controllable, hang in there Mumma as it won't be forever.

THE PLACENTA

That weird bloody thing that slops out of you post delivery. Along with your baby, inside the uterus is the placenta. An organ that is also attached to the uterine wall. The placenta is what feeds your baby nutrients & blood. The placenta also filters out unwanted waste from your babies blood as well as a number of other key things such as carbon dioxide.

On top of this, the placenta produces hormones such as progesterone & oestrogen which are essential to the mother during pregnancy. For an ugly, slippery sucker, the placenta plays a very important role in your babies life! Hence why the midwives & doctors present it to you (once you've birthed it), as if it's some kind of gourmet cuisine, procured from the depths of the Himalayan ranges. It's quite a hero in the world of baby growing. Another hero is of course the odd looking cord that hangs from the placenta.

THE UMBILICAL CORD

The umbilical cord connects the baby to the placenta,. When they say "Time to cut the cord!", it means your baby is now ready to be freed from the placenta. It's now over to Mum & Dad to take the reins!

Due to the purity & rich nutrients offered by the placenta, some women choose opt for their cord to remain connected to the baby until it naturally detaches. This is referred to by some as a Lotus Birth & it occurs when women believe their baby should have the opportunity to savor as much placenta lovin' as possible, before being swept off to a boob or a bottle. If expecting Mums are reading & thinking that this sounds lovely, be sure to do your research first as you'd need to consider that it can take up to 10days. It also means that where you and baby go … the placenta goes too.

THE CERVIX

The cervix is the area at the bottom of the uterus which sits at the top end of the vaginal canal. The cervix creates a canal between the uterus & the vagina i.e. the birth canal. During the 1st stage of labour when your cervix is dilating to 10cm, your body is preparing itself by ensuring that the opening of the birth canal is wide enough to allow your baby to move down towards your vaginal opening, closer towards the real world.

When you made it to 10cm dilated, (HOO-BLOODY-RAY!), the medical folk might have said,"your babies head is now engaged!" This meant it was go time & time for Mumma to push. From this point, with the help of hormones (the relaxin hormone in particular) both your vagina & pelvic floor muscles stretch by up to 300% of their resting length, to make room for the baby to slide down. Side Note: GO BODY GO!

THE PELVIC FLOOR

(Please read the below slowly & carefully as Pelvic Floor knowledge is critical when it comes to having babies. Due to it's importance, there is a whole chapter dedicated to learning about how to strengthen & care for your Pelvic Floor, so tools down & listen up!)

Think of your pelvic floor as a strong & very muscular pair of cupped hands. The cupped hands are in actual fact muscle and fascia, and their job (along with the help of ligament support from above), is to hold your uterus, bladder & bowel in place. In other words, the cupped hands are in charge of holding everything up & in. You with me? UP and IN.

As your baby grows and becomes heavier & heavier by the week, keeping these hands strong with a tight grip is paramount. Without strength during pregnancy, things can start to sag or droop downwards. And by things I mean organs such as your bladder & uterus. Remember how I said UP and IN earlier? Now think DOWN and OUT.

When you birth a baby vaginally (especially if you push for more than a few hours, if you required forceps or suction assistance, or if you delivered quite a big bubba), it's likely that the pelvic floor muscles will have stretched. Picture those hands coming away from each other causing their grip to loosen. This stretching can translate to weakness and this weakness can translate to sub optimal outcomes such as the loss of bladder control i.e. incontinence. The muscles in charge of controlling the bladder will have weakened leading to spontaneous wee dribbles when you sneeze, laugh or cough. Not ideal.

Worse yet, the loss of strength can cause your actual pelvic organs to sag down towards the vaginal region, causing a slight bulge or a really uncomfortable dragging sensation. Women might say their vagina feels very heavy or that their vagina feels as if it's on the verge of falling out. So forget about the UP and IN focus we went on about earlier, now think DOWN and OUT.

The DOWN and OUT debacle is what's referred to as a prolapse. What does a prolapse mean in "real terms?" Put it this way ... it means that those strong hands we've spoken about, have let a few body parts slip down & through the cracks. Basically your pelvic organs may start to protrude into the vaginal region.

The best thing you can do to avoid signs, symptoms and actual prolapse is to keep your pelvic floor strong using the help of a female physio & regular pelvic floor exercises (more on this topic coming up soon).

Let's move on from the prolapse topic for now, shall we? To make things even harder for your pelvic floor, during pregnancy a woman's body produces a series of hormones. One of which we mentioned earlier, Relaxin. The role of Relaxin is to soften a woman's ligaments, her muscles and fascia (tissue) so that a baby can comfortably grow inside of the uterus for 9 months without constriction.

Pretty cool right?!

The Relaxin hormone helps the muscles to soften so much so that a baby (or multiple babies), can beef up while continuing to fit inside of a woman's uterus. As the pelvic floor is a group of muscles, the pelvic floor softens too. Now here's the real humdinger… this new found ability to stretch isn't exactly the most helpful skill at this point in time, as for the most part we want to discourage the idea of DOWN & OUT and focus on UP & IN.

The issue with the UP and IN focus is that when a baby is delivered vaginally, Mummas pelvic floor is going to need to know how to relax so that the baby can flow out through the birth canal and safely slip into the real world to meet Mum & Dad.

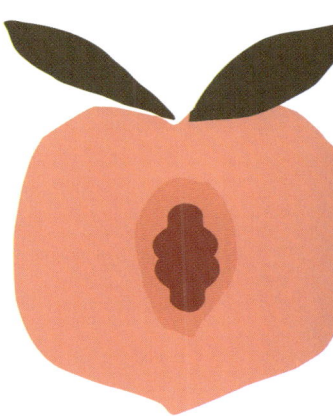

See the conundrum here? The pelvic floor needs to obey two rather contradictory commands;

Command #1) "HOLD WEES, POOS, ORGANS & BABY INSIDE UNTIL I SAY SO."

and;

Command #2) "RELEASE THE HOLD. EJECT BABY NOW!"

Sounds like a big task yes? YES it is. Again, this is why it's so important to see a women's physio throughout your pregnancy. The knowledge you'll build about your own body and the exercises you'll pick up for both birth & recovery are going to be of such value. Physios who specialise in women's health are like fairy godmothers. Wise & kind … kind being the key word.

Being kind to your body is everything!! Think of it this way. Would you play a game of tennis, sprain an ankle and then get straight back on the court? No bloody way! You would prefer to have invested in some preliminary training prior, to strengthen your ankle and avoid damage in the first place (isn't hindsight such a bitch at times!) If not, should you endure a sprain mid game, you would give yourself time & potentially rehabilitation to heal… and heal correctly.

Now where were we? Ah yes, the vagina!

THE VAGINA

Firstly of all, the vagina is not the hole where the penis & the tampon slides into. Shocked? Don't worry! I bet many people are. The vagina is a broader term for the complex area downstairs. The vagina is actually the muscular canal (i.e. the birth canal), that connects the uterus (which is of course where the baby grows), to the vulva. It's the vulva that is the hole where the penis slides into … think of it like the vaginal opening.

Side Note 1: The vaginal opening is also known as the Vestibule.

Side Note 2: Side Note 1 cracks me up!

I have no doubt there are women reading this vagina bit & already feeling a little shy or squirmy. If you're one of those women, it's fine! Human biology is not for everyone. When it comes to the vagina however, just like your knee, your nose & your hip … the vagina is another part of your body. The more you know about it, the less confusion or little surprises up ahead.

THE VULVA

To put the vulva into super simple terms and to avoid getting into too many specifics, the vulva refers to the "external bits" of your lady parts. The bits you can see in the mirror. The vulva includes the opening (aka the Vestibule), the inner & outer lips (aka the labia majora (outer lips) and the labia minora (inner lips), and the Clitoris. We good? Fab.

RECAP!

Let's have a quick drinks break & summarise what we now know;

When you birth a baby, the baby goes from…

A. The uterus (where it lives & develops for around 9 months) …

B. through the cervix (the opening of the uterus that leads to the vagina) …

C. down through the vagina (i.e. the birth canal) and;

D. out through the vulva (i.e. the vaginal opening) and into the outside world.

Hello baby! In some cases.

But what if the baby doesn't fit? This is an appropriate place to move onto The Perineum;

THE PERINEUM

The perineum is the tissue (i.e. the area of skin), in-between a woman's thighs. It sits between the vulva and the anus.

If the baby needs more space to exit the body, if the baby needs to come out quickly for medical reasons or if the baby requires assistance from forceps or suction to come out, a woman may need an episiotomy.

An episiotomy is a controlled cut into the perineum (usually on an angle to avoid the anus). An episiotomy can require stitches to repair the skin and it isn't anything to fear or loathe if you've gone through it. Tearing is, in many cases the alternative and with tearing comes less control. While tearing is still common in birth, the word control is a word we like.

An episiotomy can cause some new Mums to walk slower than a snail, sit on ice packs & have showers after going to the loo for up to 2 or more weeks. While the area will heal, the wound will be tender for sometime and must be treated carefully, kindly & hygienically to avoid infection.

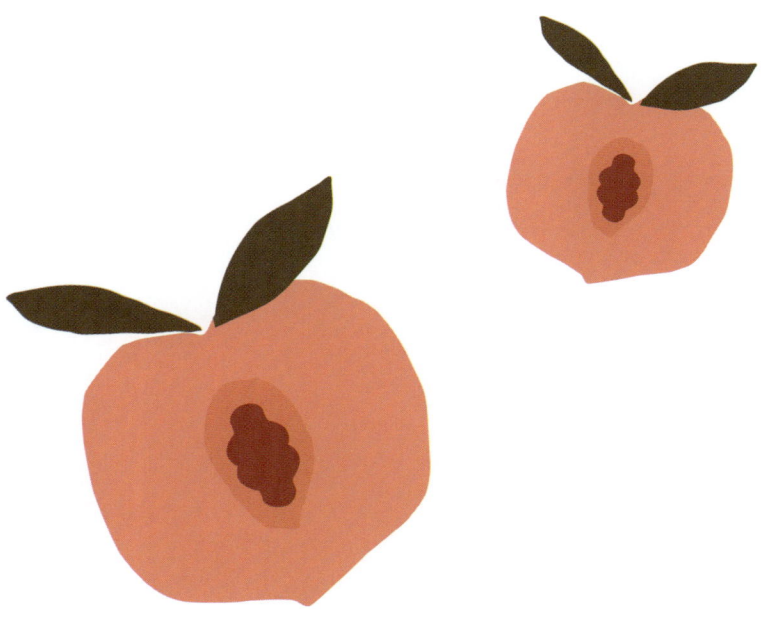

Quick Interruption! Prior to moving forward, let's invite our lovely midwife, Sophie Outhwaite to share a little more on the subject. Whether you've had an episiotomy or a tear, it is a very vulnerable & tender area of a woman's body, so it's totally natural to want to know exactly what is going on down there.

Soph, if women are too scared to get the mirror out & have a look down there after their birth but they're curious to see what's going on ... what can they expect to see? For example if they've had a tear or an episiotomy ... what does this look like/where might they expect to see the stitches?

Perineal tears range from 1st degree involving only perineal skin, to the most severe 4th degree tears which involve perineal skin, perineal muscles and the internal and external anal sphincter. If you had an episiotomy, whoever cut it likely did so medio-laterally (on a 45 degree angle, away from the anus – if you can picture that).

Whatever injury you had would likely have been neatly sutured up, either in the delivery room by your midwife or doctor, or (often in the case of 3rd and 4th degree tears) in theatre. Swelling and small amounts of bleeding are normal and should decrease with time. Your vagina might also be wider (of course!) but this should start to reduce a few days after your baby is born.

Do you recommend having a look with a mirror? Or should women give it 6 weeks to let it heal before seeing something they can't "un-see"?

Your imagination is probably worse than the reality. I think it is a good idea to know what your wound looks like. That way you can track improvement: your perineum should heal like other wounds, gradually becoming less sore, less red and less swollen.

Moving forwards, the anus.

THE ANUS

The bum, the toosh, the buttocks. The poop hole. Enough said? Ok good.

Speaking of the anus, if you are worried you poo'd during birth, don't sweat it! It's a sign you pushed into the right area and a sign you're human. You pooped before having your baby and you'll poo after. It's ok.

THE BLADDER

The bladder is of course the organ that holds your urine. The bladder is a hollow organ held in place by ligaments i.e. connective tissues that hold internal structures together. As the baby grows in the uterus, the growing uterus can push into the bladder causing pregnant women to feel as if they need to pee far more frequently than usual … even when their bladder is far less than full.

THE URETHRA

The wee hole.

Ok so before we move onto new topics, let's just circle back to a topic that many readers are probably still sweating over.

PROLAPSE

To quickly refresh… what is prolapse? Prolapse or Pelvic Organ Prolapse (POP), is a common condition affecting 50% of parous women (that is, women who have had babies), and 40% of women over the age of 50.

POP is the descent of any pelvic organ (bladder, uterus, rectum or bowel) into the vagina, or beyond the vagina introitus (the exterior side of the vaginal opening). The presence of a vaginal lump or bulge is the most specific sign correlated with a prolapse, however you can prevent it!!

Simple Steps To Reduce The Risk Of Prolapse ...

While it's not uncommon to experience partial prolapse post birth, meaning you might only encounter few or faint symptoms, it's important to do whatever necessary to avoid any level of prolapse. Prevention is the best cure!

- It's highly recommended that you see a trusted a women's health physio before you become pregnant, during your pregnancy & most definitely after you deliver! This advice goes for all women regardless of age, fitness & general health. A women's health physio will identify your individual risk factors & manage your downstairs region accordingly.

Please Note that Google is not a physio. Every single woman is physically different, so caring for your pelvic floor is not necessarily a case of one size fits all.

- Avoid unnecessary straining on the toilet. If you're backed up, look into managing constipation & keep yourself very well hydrated (especially if you're breastfeeding).

- Stay on top of your appropriate exercises during pregnancy & postpartum. Your physio will create the exercise regime for you.

- Don't over do it! When you come home from the hospital, avoid too many long walks, heavy lifting (including toddlers where possible), and squatting. Lay down and give your pelvic floor a change to heal and recover. You can suffer from prolapse during the postpartum period (or any stage of life for that matter). It is not something that occurs solely due to pregnancy & birth.

How will you know if you have a prolapse (or a partial prolapse)?

◊ If you notice a lump or a bulge in the vagina or on the outside.

◊ If you feel a noticeable heaviness or a dragging sensation during the day or after you exercise.

◊ If your vagina aches.

◊ If you notice any changes to your regular bladder and/or bowel movements.

If you do notice any of the above, your women's physio can accurately and safely grade the level of prolapse and treat you accordingly. To reiterate the point above, this is not a "one size fits all" issue. Every single woman is built differently.

THE WHOLE BODY NIGHT SWEATS

One of the biggest postpartum surprises may be the night sweats, (it was for me!). Waking up drenched in sweat, even during the cooler months, is horrendous. It can be especially hard to cope with when you throw leaking breastmilk into the mix.

The night sweats can be the result of a few factors such as your hormone levels. As your body readjusts its levels of oestrogen and progesterone post birth, the temperature of your body is also likely to change and cool off. Remember how warm you felt while you were pregnant?

Another common reason for postpartum night sweats is that your body is getting rid of excess fluids. While women are pregnant, they carry more blood than usual. After birthing their baby the body reabsorbs the blood & it can be excreted in sweat & pee.

SUMMARY OF THE BODY

Ok so now we should have a basic idea of what's what. If you're even more curious and you'd like to learn more, Phoebe Marinovich, our adored resident women's health physio, can be found at @f_e_m_m_e___silasphysio. Follow along & indulge in her knowledge and brilliance!

Phoebe encourages women to grab a mirror and take a quick peak downstairs. Using the mirror can help create a positive relationship between a woman & her vagina so she never feels detached from it or fearful of it.

From safety point of view, familiarising yourself with your own vagina is also a good idea as it'll help you pick up on any changes. If you notice that something doesn't look or feel quite right, you should always seek medical advice.

2 FINAL THINGS!

Before we end The Body chapter we better touch on two final elements to do with the upstairs region.

HAIR

… or the loss of it postpartum.

Firstly, we can't talk about hair and fail to acknowledge how wonderful pregnancy hair is. That would just be rude! For some women, their pregnancy hair is thick, glossy, strong & buoyant. It's a treat and it definitely makes up for a few of the not so glamorous things women endure for 9 months (such as the need to pee thirteen times per night).

We can thank the heightened levels of oestrogen for these lovely thick locks! What's crazy is that your body isn't actually growing more hair, but it's just that your hair is growing at a faster rate (hence the extra length you notice), and you are losing less hair at a slower rate. How great!

Postpartum hair is a little different.

In the 6 or so months after delivering, it's very common for women to lose hair & and in some unfortunate cases, a lot of it. Some women will experience whole clumps falling out in the shower or notice a heap of strands on their pillow in the morning. Sound distressing? I'd say so! If this is you, don't feel as though you are being shallow because your insecurities are having a field day due to the thickness of your hair. If you feel panicked and down about it, your feelings are wholeheartedly valid and shared by SO many women!

Just as hormones affect the thickness & length of your locks during pregnancy, hormones also happen to be the culprit behind hair loss when the baby arrives. There is a big decline in your oestrogen levels which triggers your body to get back to the normal hair shedding routine. Rather than losing the normal 80 or so strands of hair per day during the postpartum period women can lose up to 400 strands per day! So if you think you're going crazy…you're not! Those clumps or bald spots are not in your imagination!

To explain the rapid loss in simple terms, your head is playing catch up. All of the hair that it "held onto" during pregnancy now needs to come out (sadly). So out it comes with quite a force.

Again, if this makes you feel self conscious, it's ok. Despite hair loss being so common during postpartum (not all women will experience it), it doesn't make it an easier pill to swallow. The good news? Your hair should return to normal around month six. If you were hoping the words month six was a typo and it should've say week, regrettably it was not. Hang in there!!

There are SO many amazing haircare products and supplements on the market that can help to soften the hair loss blow! Dry up your tears & chat to your girlfriends or your hairdresser. You'll be amazed at what you can find.

SKIN

This won't be a long spiel as the subject of skin and skincare is so complex as it's completely unique to each and every person on this planet, regardless of whether or not they've had a baby.

People's skin type and the condition of their skin it heavily related to genetics, hormones, age, lifestyle and a whole range of other external factors such as the weather. Skin is not something that can or should be generalised as it's a convoluted cluster of factors. So leading people, especially new Mummas, to think otherwise can often bring on stress & maybe even unwanted inflammation.

For this reason we'll focus on a range of conditions that may appear during the pregnancy & postpartum period. To do this, we're very lucky to welcome the wonderful skin specialist, Natalie Beaumont. Natalie has not only shed some light on very common wonders & worries but she's listed a whole bunch of dynamite advice to help the health of our complexion. Enjoy!

1. During pregnancy a flood of hormones rushes through the female body & it can send the skin into a tizz! Common conditions include Pregnancy Acne, Melasma and Hyperpigmentation. Can you explain each of these in simple terms?

Yes for sure!

Acne: During the first and second trimester, your hormones are in overdrive, namely progesterone, and this hormone can increase sebaceous gland activity (oil) and inflammation in the skin - leading to breakouts. It's commonly experienced around the chin and jawline.

Melasma: A hormonal pigmentation that presents as darker patches of skin, and can appear symmetrical on both sides of face. This is sometimes referred to as the "pregnancy mask". The forehead, the tops of cheeks and the upper lip are commonly affected areas. This is due to the spike in hormones which stimulate the melanocytes (pigment producing cells). Some women are more genetically predisposed to this.

Pigmentation: While not all women will experience Melasma, most will notice a darkening of their existing freckles, and will notice their skin is more sensitive to the sun throughout pregnancy. Other areas that may darken are the nipples, as well as a darker line that runs down the centre of your belly, called linea nigra. This darkening generally fades back to pre-pregnancy colour as your hormones settle postpartum.

2. In terms of skincare products, during pregnancy & when women breastfeed, they're told not to use Vitamin A and Retinol. Why is this and when they be reintroduced?

During pregnancy and breastfeeding, women are advised to not use certain ingredients on their skin. The two most common ingredients are Salicylic acid (BHA) and Retinol (vitamin A). This is due to potential toxicity to the fetus. It should be noted that this is the case when either of these ingredients are taken orally (i.e. such as salicylic acid - aspirin, Vitamin A - accutane).

No studies have been done to show adverse effects when either are applied topically, however most women still choose to avoid them while pregnant or breastfeeding.

Low dose Salicylic of 2% is considered safe and very effective when applied topically for skin suffering breakouts throughout pregnancy.

There are also some skincare ranges which use a natural alternative to Retinol, called Bakuchiol, as well as Retinyl Palmitate. Most topical retinols in skincare are not able to penetrate into the bloodstream, therefore they can be considered safe. This is a personal choice yet it is always recommended you talk to your individual health care provider before taking or applying anything to make an informed decision.

3. Sun sensitivity is quite prominent during pregnancy & the postpartum period. Why is this?

Throughout pregnancy, your skin may feel more sensitive in general, but also particularly to the sun. This is due to (again!) the rise in hormones, a higher volume of blood (which raises your body temperature), and a lowered immune system.

Your pigment producing cells are also stimulated, so you will be especially susceptible to more freckling and darker patches of skin.

The areas where the skin stretches (belly, boobs, hips, bum) are the areas more sensitive to sun exposure, so it's important to be diligent with your sunscreen and reapplying when exposed to the sun. A high protection broad spectrum sunscreen is recommended, and if your skin feels more sensitive or reactive, look for zinc based sunscreens.

4. If during either pregnancy or breastfeeding women notice intense patchiness in their skin-tone, is there anything they can introduce to help with this?

While this is usually a hormonally driven aspect, and can sometimes fade of its own accord when your hormones revert back to their regular levels, there is certainly no harm in using skincare to help this process along.

Pregnancy safe brightening ingredients include:

- ◊ Vitamin C
- ◊ Licorice
- ◊ Azelaic acid
- ◊ Niacinamide (B3)
- ◊ Lactic/Glycolic/Mandelic acids (Alpha Hydroxy Acids - AHAs)

Gentle exfoliation using a chemical exfoliant like the above AHAs, can help with brightening the skins appearance. This can be done twice a week with a low percentage AHA. They can come in the form of toners, serums, swipey soaked cotton pads.

A good quality serum with a blend of the above ingredients applied daily to help tackle existing pigmentation, as well as preventing further overproduction of pigment.

Also SUNSCREEN!!!! There is no point applying all your serums and brighteners if you are not going to religiously use and reapply your sunscreen everyday to protect your skin!!

And finally;

5. What key ingredients are fantastic for easy, nourishing and hydrating skincare. When newborns are taking up so much of the day, it's nice to have a few go-to products that women don't have to think too much about. Any recommendations?

With a newborn, there is very little time or craving for an elaborate skincare routine. However, if you can steal 1-2 minutes to yourself in the mornings and evenings for a bit of self care, your skin will love you for it.

In the postpartum period, your skin is likely to be more dehydrated, so ingredients to look out for to combat this are

Hyaluronic acid, Ceramides and Omega 3 fatty acids.

A vitamin C serum will help with "perking" your skin up. Vitamin C will also feed your skin with antioxidants and help to treat discolouration.

An all in one moisturiser and sunscreen with high SPF will be a great multitasking product for you. Some formulas are tinted, which can be great if you want a little coverage during the day.

An example of a quick & simple daily routine could be something like the following;

MORNING:

- A gentle face cloth (flannel) can be used in the mornings with warm or cool water (not hot!)
- Brightening antioxidant serum applied - go for a hydrating formula.
- Hydrating moisturiser with SPF 30 at minimum.

EVENING:

- A mild cleanser massaged in to the skin and removed with soft wash cloth.
- A hyaluronic serum
- Nourishing moisturiser

Extra Tips: Keep your products where they are easily accessible to you eg: put your moisturiser next to your bed or where you breastfeed or pump.

AFTERWARDS

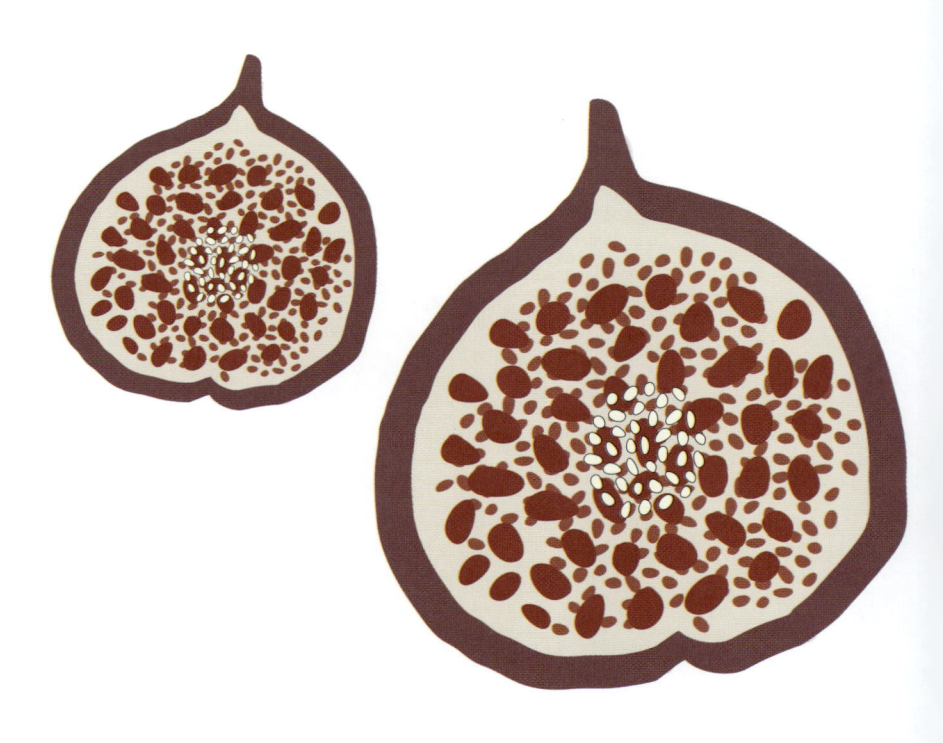

Before we finish up on the topic of skincare, our midwife Sophie Outhwaite has added a few additional comments & insights that are definitely worth reading if you're still wondering why you're not advised to take or use certain products while pregnant or breastfeeding;

In general, pregnant women & breastfeeding Mummas have to be hyper aware of any medications they take & skincare they use. For those who don't take this too seriously - can you briefly explain the implications of exposing the body to particular ingredients?

Research into medication safety during pregnancy is complicated by a number of factors. Basically, the research is hard to do. Because of the lack of data supporting safety of medications, it is wise to err on the side of caution: don't take anything you don't need to, and always talk to your doctor or pharmacist first.

In Australia, legal drugs are classified by the Therapeutic Goods Authority (TGA) on the safety of drugs during pregnancy. These classifications have been developed by scientific experts based on the available evidence of risks associated with taking particular drugs during pregnancy. When prescribing medications, health professionals consider these classifications.

Be aware that most medicines cross the placenta. The TGA's categorisation system takes into account the known harmful effects of medications on the developing baby, including the potential to cause birth defects, unwanted pharmacological effects around the time of birth and problems for the baby later in life.

Letters to myself...

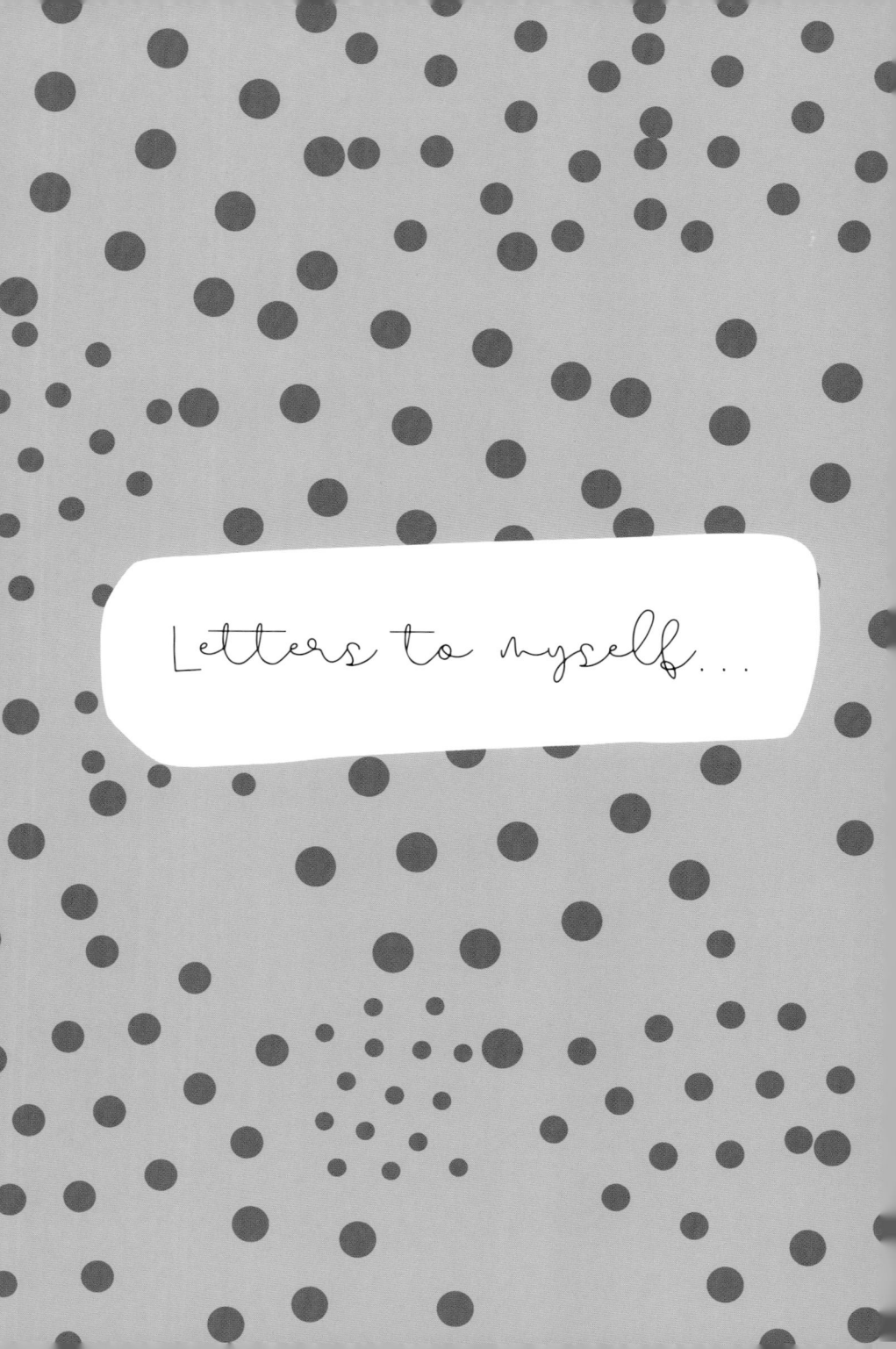

Dear me,

... the side of myself that is always asking, is this "new normal" what you wanted?

Yes it is. It might not always mimic what I expected in particular moments, but it is.

It makes me feel tired. I'm coping however I am without my bearings. Is it Tuesday? Is it Friday? Is it noon or first light? While I might sound lost on a timeline, please don't fret as I have everything I need in my arms. This little being I hold, we hold, is actually quite heavy ... oh, so heavy in fact. Do you agree? Despite my lethargic limbs I will keep my grip firm. So yes. I am tired, it is true - but I am ok. I might look pale or flushed but I am green with the opposite of envy as you'll find that I am content. And, I am stronger than I've ever felt before. Don't worry about me, about us. They call us a mother now & this lovely new title is our armour, our coat. My will, your fortune. Our all. I will feel fine when the coffee is poured & the toast is buttered. Just dim the light for now and let my eyes rest and my chest seek respite. I will find you in the morning and I will make sure not to push you too hard. We shall rise & smile together, for tomorrow is another day in our paradise. Our loud, our own, our prized paradise. x

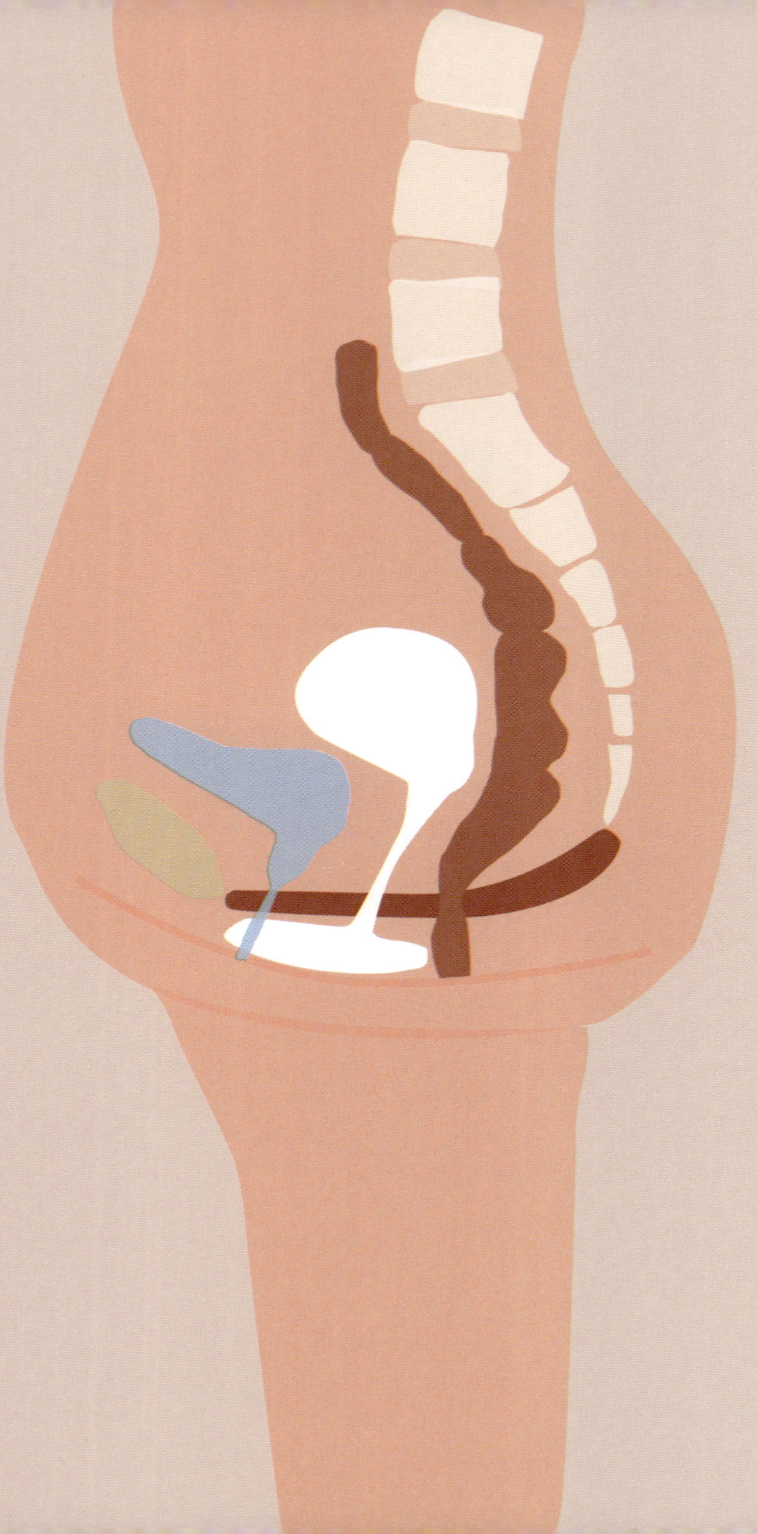

CHAPTER 2

the pelvic floor

Spinal Cord

Uterus

Bladder

Pubic Bone

Anus

Pelvic Floor

P 54　AFTERWARDS

LET'S RECAP. WHAT IS THE PELVIC FLOOR?

The pelvic floor consists of muscles & fascia (i.e. connecting tissue) located inside of the pelvis. The pelvis is a complex of bones that connects your trunk to your legs.

The pelvic floor muscles is a group of muscles that sit like a hammock at the base of your pelvis. They work to keep us continent (in terms of both our bladder and bowel), they support the pelvic organs (i.e. the bladder, bowel & uterus), and they support the lumbar spine with the lower abdominals. Finally, the pelvic floor muscles support sexual function. They are very important in terms of arousal and climax.

Now let's go over the role of the pelvic floors during pregnancy & after pregnancy? And how it works in relation to the uterus & the vagina.

During pregnancy there is a lot of added pressure and weight on the pelvic floor due to the baby growing inside of the uterus. From the size of a blueberry, they grow into a melon before you know it! Due to the growing weight, the pelvic floor muscles have to work harder than ever to keep us continent, and to support the pelvic organs.

As we spoke about in The Body chapter, the hormonal effect of pregnancy (particularly the addition of the relaxin hormone), causes our ligaments, our fascia and our muscles to soften in preparation for the birth. The softening effect also occurs to accommodate the baby in the uterus. With all of this in mind, during pregnancy a woman's pelvic floor needs to perform!

After the baby is born, the pelvic floor muscles are not off the hook just yet. They're required to get back to work asap. Back they go to holding everything UP and IN. As the pelvic floor has been working over time during the 9 month pregnancy, it's not uncommon for the pelvic floor to be tired and weak.

Anyone finding themselves weeing a little when they cough, laugh or sneeze? If so, this is a classic example of the pelvic floor lacking the strength to retain full control.

For this reason, women really need to add some extra TLC into their day to ensure they regain their strength asap post birth. Particularly for women who would like to have more babies. If you can prioritise and nail a full or at least a decent recovery, your body will cope much better when it's time to grow and birth another baby, compared to if you became complacent after baby #1.

The best way to regain strength and control? Exercise!

Gentle exercises post birth can be great when practiced correctly and regularly. Generally speaking it should be ok to commence some gentle exercises straight after birth, as long your catheter is out. However before launching in, it's absolutely encouraged to get the official OK from your maternal health nurse, your GP or your women's health physio.

Before we explore some exercises, let's address a very common question;"How long will it take my Pelvic Floor to recover post birth?"

This is the million dollar question & unfortunately one with no definitive answer. Your recovery time will depend on a number of varying factors, including of course your genetics, your pregnancy & your birth.

- ◊ Those who endured a traumatic delivery may encounter a decent amount of swelling, bruising or even more severe damage. This can take some time to heal & these women might be a little late returning to the trampoline.

- ◊ Those who are genetically blessed & have very elastic, stretchy skin around their downstairs region may bounce back a little sooner.

- ◊ Those who are diligent & committed to practising regular pelvic floor exercises & prioritise visits with their women's health physio may notice an accelerated recovery time as well. Working with a women's health physio is an incredible way to receive guided feedback regarding your body. It's important to remember that matters of the pelvic floor are unique to each individual. What you require is not what they require.
- ◊ Those who suffered a prolapse post birth or a partial prolapse may encounter a slightly more uphill battle in terms of their recovery as their set back is a little more complex.

This list could go on but it's best not to fuel your mind with worries & override positive thinking. Especially as it's never too late to strengthen your pelvic floor. You are not broken. The life & times of your vagina does not have to be defined by your choice to be a mother. But try and surrender to the fact that it takes time, work (and rest), patience & self awareness.

As mentioned, there are so many contributing factors to the recovery of a woman's pelvic floor after birth. As you're on the road to recovery, remember that even though your stitches may have dissolved & your vagina appears to be less swollen, never discount what is going on internally.

Birth doesn't just affect the side we can see. The birth canal, the uterus, the bladder … all of these internal parts of your body have gone through a hell of a time. They'll be bruised and tender at the very least, so go easy on yourself. Show your body the respect it deserves & in due course it'll return the favour.

Before we move onto exercises, make sure to remind yourselves that pelvic floor health & strength is not only related to pregnancy and birth. It's an area of your body that requires focus & attention at all times, for both females and males.

THE KEGAL

The Kegal is an exercise that works the pelvic floor muscles. It's almost like a "vaginal squeeze".

First up; the best way to ensure you're exercising the right area is to make sure nobody can detect you're doing your kegals when you're doing them! If your buttocks and thighs are lifting, you're not using the right muscles.

How To Kegal;

- ◊ Imagine you are sitting on a small marble ball & you are trying to lift the marble up using your vagina. Another thought, imagine there is a straw in your vagina and you're using it to suck liquids upwards.
- ◊ As you feel the upwards squeeze, now imagine as if you're simultaneously trying to hold in wind.
- ◊ Identify this feeling as you squeeze, hold & release.
- ◊ As well as your buttocks and thighs, nothing higher than your belly button should move or contract while doing your Kegals. And avoid holding your breath!

How Many & How Often?

- Hold each Kegal for 3-10 seconds & repeat them 5-10times.

- In the very early postpartum days when you're still recovering, be very gentle & take it slowly. It's always recommended that you check with your midwife, maternal health nurse or women's health physio before commencing your vaginal workout.

- Aim for a few sets per day. A nice way to remember to do your exercises is to do them while doing another daily task, such as taking a shower. If it becomes associated to an existing routine you are much less likely to forget.

If you had been practising daily Kegals before and during your pregnancy (first of all, good on you!), you may notice that following your birth the exercise might feel quite different & quite possibly more difficult. This is normal.

The muscles will be fatigued & slightly weaker due to the pregnancy and birth. Do your best to solider on with your Kegals though, as it'll assist with the healing process and it might even help to reduce swelling.

WARNING

Practising Kegals while doing a wee (i.e. by trying to stop your wee mid-stream is not advised). The "wee test" is not a good habit to fall into as it can create negative bladder habits.

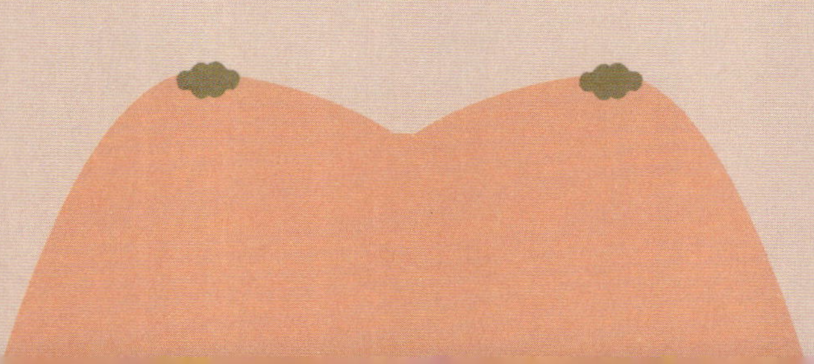

CHAPTER 3

boobs

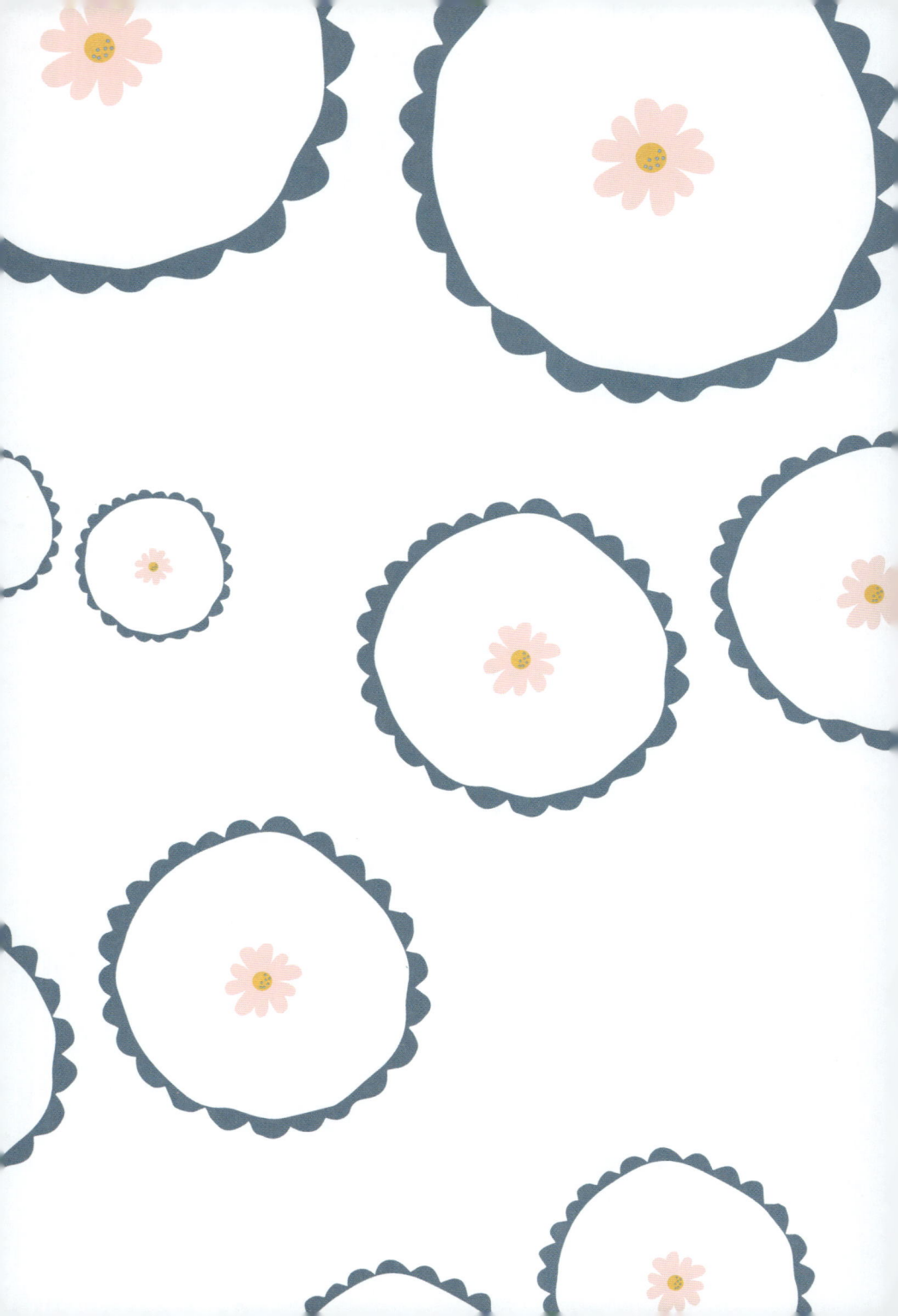

Is it day 3, 4, or 5 and you're home from the hospital with your beautiful baby? Did you wake up this morning, look down and think to yourself ... "What In Gods Name Are Those?"

I Hear You. Does it look like the world's most botched boob job has crawled into your home & ever so comfortably made itself at home on your chest?

If this sounds like your situation, trust me when I say that when your midwife or your maternal health nurse visits you next, they will celebrate & proudly tell you, "How fabulous! Your milk has come in!"

While they celebrate your new assets, you'll probably sweat in mortified shock horror. "I asked for a child. Not a Z cup that hits my chin & sits under my armpits."

The early days of your milk supply, especially if it leads to engorgement, can be a somewhat hard adjustment (pardon the very fitting pun here). If you had quite a small cup size prior to falling pregnant, your eyes might fall out of their sockets every morning as it really is a peculiar sight.

Does it look or feel sexy? Ummm? Not so much. If your partner seems excited by your new astronomical pair of boobs, ask them how they'd feel if you slipped an uber strong viagra into their drink & followed that up by using a pump to inflate their penis until it was on the cusp of bursting. It ain't sexy when it aches.

The good news? Your baby's tucker has just arrived.

Your boobs are in many ways a part of your femininity. Maybe not for all, but for many. You buy them pretty bras & fancy crops to push them up & perkify them. You cater to their every need pending the activities for the day. At the gym, you make sure they're dressed to fight the painful bounce. When it's cold you layer up to avoid "stiffles". When you hit the beach you pander to their tanning needs by amending your straps. And when you are totally exhausted and you can't work out why the Vegemite is under the bathroom sink, you pour a glass of wine, tie a topknot & remove your bra, freeing your boobs from the underwire that restricts their daily freedom.

The things we do for our boobs! And rightly so as they absolutely deserve the TLC. We owe a lot to them.

Boobs can fire up that sexy feeling & take sex from a 5 to a 10. Boobs can make an outfit … and let's be honest here, they can break an outfit just as quickly. Boobs can ignite a sense of pride and womanhood as they grow & change with your developing shape. Your boobs are a powerhouse! Best yet, if you are lucky they can allow you to feed your baby.

Breastfeeding, should you go down the breastfeeding path, can be a prickly affair until you & bub find your rhythm. Finding your rhythm may take days, weeks, or even months, so if you relate to the latter it's nothing to lose sleep over.

Breastfeeding is not as easy as we all assumed when observing other mothers do it so intuitively. It's a fidgety activity that might cause frustration, irritation, and impatience. It might cause pain & discomfort. It might cause tears and a sense of failure. But it should never push you to doubt yourself as a Mum. The only personal tip I'll throw in while we're on the topic of breastfeeding (I'm sure you've all been flooded with millions of annoying tips by now!), but … imagine your boob is a whopping hamburger. To bite this hamburger and get all the layers in one mouthful, you need to squish it down using your hands. Apply this same idea to your full boob & try to use your hands to create an area that is easier for the baby's mouth to get around.

If all else fails and you feel like you may implode, grab a bottle. It is not a crime. It's a feed.

Let's go back a step though. Before the feeding begins, we can't pretend like the 9 months of pregnancy didn't bring along a string of boob changes.

As soon as you see those two pink lines appear on the pregnancy stick, your boobs start to stack on a few. It's as if they're bulking for a starring role in a superhero film! They get bigger, they feel heavier & for some women, stretch marks or rivers of veins appear as if flood gates have just opened. In the early days of pregnancy, your boobs might ache obnoxiously, making sleep interrupted and uncomfortable. Even a tight hug from a friend can bring water to the eye.

And the nipples?! Why doesn't anyone warn you about the isolated nipple pain! On a cold or a windy day as your body shivers in the chill, it can feel as if shards of glass are cutting through your top & biting down on your nipples. You have to hold on & apply firm pressure to numb this painful sting.

The boobs really do take a hit as they prepare for their next role in life; The Human Smorgasbord. And it doesn't end here.

Let's talk about The Leaking. Oh sweet Moses, The Leaking.

LEAKING

It's wild but so true that a woman's boobs may leak colostrum during pregnancy. Women and their organisation skills right?! Even their bodies are one step ahead of the game, stocking up the fridge before the guest of honour arrives. Leaking isn't the end of the world (who doesn't love stuffing toilet paper or panty liners in their bra when a boob starts to dribble), but just when women are able to take a 9 month holiday from their monthly period, what, another leak springs? Is it really too much to ask for the female body to just turn off all taps for a small window of time? Is it really?!

Oh, boobs! Boobs, boobs, boobs.

When your baby finally arrives, this is the time when the boobs really get to work. It's their time to shine baby! For many women (not all, which is totally fine!), your boobs become your baby's breakfast, lunch, dinner, midnight feast & hourly snack. Your boobs become your babies teething toy, their pillow, their comforter, their portable cot.

You don't dress your boobs in pretty bras anymore … you coat them in armour. Nipple pads, thick layers of paw paw ointment or Lanolin, and maternity bras that are more robust than a bulletproof vest. Some may even choose to dress their boobs in frozen cabbage leaves resulting in a smell that can only be compared to the thing dying at the bottom of your fridge.

You'll have days where you feel really womanly & lovely in your newfound shape. You might even feel confident and super sexy! On other days, especially the early days when your milk comes in, you'll look in the mirror & think to yourself, "Why do they look SO ANGRY at me?"

If this is you today, don't fret! Your boobs will eventually soften & once again find their smile. They'll graciously build a friendship with your baby and proceed to generously feed and nourish their bellies, allowing a bond that is sweet & instinctive.

When your milk has come in & the feeding train has left the station, your boobs will start their round-the-clock shift work. The left boob feeds & then clocks off. The right boob feeds & then clocks off. And so the cycle continues. Emptying one boob before offering the other is commonly recommended as it can help women to avoid blocked ducts. If you're nervous about forgetting which boob you're up to, there are plenty of apps to keep a digital boob diary such as Baby Tracker. There is an app for everything regarding newborns and babies … e v e r y t h i n g.

Keeping on top of your boobs is a good habit to fall into from the get-go as I'd say all women will agree that avoiding blocked ducts & worse yet, avoiding mastitis (aka The Boob Flu), is the goal.

MASTITIS

According to the Australian Breastfeeding Association, mastitis is usually the result of a blocked milk duct that hasn't cleared. Some of the milk banked up behind the blocked duct can be forced into nearby breast tissue, causing the tissue to become inflamed. The inflammation is called mastitis & in some cases, it may be partnered with a pretty vicious infection.

Sound horrible? I think so too.

If you are just starting your breastfeeding journey & you're curious about mastitis warning signs, it's best to look out for these common symptoms:

- ◊ Fever
- ◊ Whole Body Chills
- ◊ Body Aches
- ◊ Feeling Tired and Lethargic
- ◊ Exceptionally Tender or Warm Boobs
- ◊ Feeling Generally Unwell

So that's mastitis! Let's take a second to move onto our mate The Pump.

THE PUMP

The Pump represents a love-hate relationship. In so many ways it's a lifesaver. In so many other ways it's a time consuming, uncomfortable hindrance & hooking yourself up to it can make you feel pretty low & pretty yuck.

Let's start with the positive. Why do we love The Pump?

- ◊ It can relieve so much pressure on the boobs when they're full to the brim & when you're not in the position to feed your baby. If the baby is asleep or if you're at work or attending a social function, not having the option to drain your swollen, heavy boobs is very uncomfortable. Not only does it feel uncomfortable but as your boobs grow into rock hard melons you may feel a little self-conscious as your cleavage is now all of a sudden on show. If you have a vast difference in supply from right to left… you may get a few odd looks!

- ◊ If your bubba is having trouble with the latch or if you're yet to find a rhythm and your baby is crying for a feed the marriage between the pump and the bottle is a great solution. I repeat … the pump + the bottle is a great solution. If The Pump isn't an option & there is formula in the cupboard … the bottle + the formula is another GREAT solution as #FEDISBEST

- ◊ If your baby is tongue-tied and therefore isn't able to adequately extract enough milk with their suck.

- ◊ If you have inverted nipples & need the pump to help shape your nipple.

- ◊ If you choose not to breastfeed as you prefer the idea of expressing milk with the pump & feeding the baby with a bottle.

- ◊ It's a fabulous accessory. I mean who doesn't love pairing a new dress & heels with an electronic, double pump monstrosity with suction cups the size of drink bottles?

For the reasons above, The Pump is our mate.

From another perspective, however, The Pump can feel like a little bitch.

◊ When it's 7pm and you've just put the baby down. You're ready for a shower, a wine, bed, or simply a conversation with another adult aged human … and then you remember… you have to milk yourself.

◊ If you have an oversupply of milk & therefore you need to pump after every feed. You feel robbed of downtime & stuck on your bum again.

◊ The Pump can make you feel like an animal. Some may argue with this and that's totally fine, but pumping can make you feel as if you've morphed into a dairy cow.

◊ Pumping offers yet another point of comparison. Your girlfriend might have a freezer full of expressed breastmilk (EMB), yet you've only collected 65ml (between BOTH boobs), after 45 minutes. You feel inept, shitty and empty. Literally.

◊ Pumping can lead to spillage. Imagine after those 45minutes you stand up & accidentally spill one or both of the pump bottles, losing all of your EBM. A river of tears doesn't fall from your eyes … an almighty tidal wave oozes from every orifice in your body. And finally;

◊ It's another goddam charger to pack when you go away.

So yes, The Pump is an amazing gadget & one that comes highly recommended by midwives & so many other mothers. But if you're someone who truly feels stuck, bored, ugly, and plain old cow-like when you're using your pump be assured there are others just like you.

SHAPE & SIZE

Boobs are quite a significant part of a woman's body whether they're an A Cup or an F Cup. Whether they're a natural pair, a reduced pair, an implanted pair, or perhaps they're now two healing scars. Boobs take the female kind from girl, to teen, to woman, to mother. They are unique as no pair is the same and they're ever-changing.

When your weight changes, they change. When your period arrives, they change. When your age ticks over to another year, they change. When your hormones dance or cry, they change. When you're pregnant, they change. When you breastfeed, they change. When you stop breastfeeding, they change. Not only that, but some sets of boobs change at different rates. Anyone else look drastically lopsided when they first wake up in the morning while breastfeeding? Holy hell is that sight a rude awaking.

For those reading who endured months of radically misshaped boobs due to a significant difference in milk supply from left to right, I hear you Mumma! I'm honestly surprised I didn't develop a limp as I lugged my giant right boob around for almost 12months.

The difference in milk supply from right to left can occur for a number of reasons. Your milk ducts may differ side to side, your letdown might be more forceful on one side or perhaps you prefer to feed on one particular boob. The supply can be affected if you've suffered an illness or undergone surgery or one boob might just like to put her feet up and chill the hell out! Regardless of the reason the misshaped boob affair is another weird & wonderful postpartum occurrence. You're not a freak show. You're a great Mum.

If you want to try & even them out there are some recommend ways to encourage the milk supply on a particular side. A few examples include:

- ◊ Pumping on the slower side for a little longer than the other
- ◊ Starting a feed on the least preferred side
- ◊ Hand massage or expressing milk in the shower

Speaking of size, let's talk implants.

IMPLANTS

I think it's so important to highlight & draw focus to Mummas who have had breast augmentation & go onto having a baby who they choose to breastfeed. Maybe it's just me but I feel as though you don't hear an awful lot about the subject of breastfeeding with implants & I'd say it's safe to assume that women with implants are more curious than they may let on. Totally understandable.

To answer a few common questions and wondering thoughts on the issue, we have the lovely Sarah Mitchell. Sarah is the nurse to a highly regarded surgeon in Australia & she's generously shared some of her excellent and comforting wisdom with us.

1. Can you breastfeed with implants?

Absolutely! Implants are usually placed in a dual plane (most of the implant is behind the muscle, a small amount of the implant is intact with the skin on the lower 1/3). This means that it does not sit on milk ducts and/or interfere with your body's ability to produce milk and/or breastfeed. However, there are SOME women that are naturally not able to breastfeed (usually those with Tuberous breast deformities). These women will still not be able to breastfeed.

Patients who have a breast lift with implants will have some of their milk ducts removed in the process of removing excess skin to reshape the breast. A good surgeon will try to keep most of the ducts intact, so as to not interfere with their ability to breastfeed. However, we always tell our patients they are approximately 30% - 70% less likely to be able to breastfeed after this surgery.

2. In layman's terms can you explain the difference of how a boob without implants operates in terms of producing milk, VS how a boob with implants does? Or is there no difference?

No difference.

3. For women using an electric pump, are there any precautions they should take? For example, should they be using a lower/slower setting when pumping?

Definitely a slower setting. Most patients with implants won't feel comfortable using a pump. From my understanding the breast pump is quite traumatic to the skin meaning the Mum will be more prone to excess skin (which will change the appearance of the breast).

4. If there was an issue (lack of milk, pain, engorgement, swelling, nipple irritation or loss of feeling, etc), how would a woman know if the issue is related to her implants or if it's simply to do with her natural milk supply?

It is really important for Mums who have breast implants to be aware of changes to their breasts throughout the pregnancy and breastfeeding journey. We usually recommend patients to have scans (Ultrasound and/or MRI scanning - NOT mammogram) if they are having issues with their breasts before/during their pregnancy. They do this to check the integrity of the implants to ensure there are no ruptures/ leaks. If there is a rupture we say not to breastfeed as we don't really know what will be transferred to the baby.

The biggest concern would be if the Mum develops mastitis. This is caused by blocked milk ducts and usually requires antibiotic therapy. Mums without breast implants can often massage this (if caught early) and be given other techniques (not antibiotics) to reduce the incidence and symptoms. However Mums with implants that develop this are at very high risk of developing Capsular Contracture (scar tissue that develops around the breast implant distorting the shape and causing hardening). With this in mind, those that develop symptoms of mastitis should start antibiotic therapy sooner rather than later.

When pregnant or new Mums call up and ask me this question we recommend they have an ultrasound (under the guidance of their OBGYN or midwife).

5. For women with implants, who is the best person to talk to about any issues with boobs post-birth, pain, or discomfort for women breastfeeding with implants? Should they call their cosmetic surgeon or their obstetrician/midwife?

Usually their OBGYN or their midwife. But if they are having ongoing swelling or discomfort, definitely their surgeon.

6. Bra wise, what is the recommended type of bra for implants? Traditional nursing bras? No underwire? Tight/loose/no bra?

Good supportive bras. This helps to reduce the chance of developing excess skin post breastfeeding and is best for the aesthetics following. Underwire bras are great, very supportive and if fitted correctly should sit just below the implant. We actually tell our patients to wear underwire bras from 2-3 weeks post-operatively.

7. Same question as above, but in terms of sleep. What should women with implants (who are breastfeeding), wear to bed for both comfort & boob support?

Their post-operative compression bra is great if they still have it. Otherwise a tight-fitting crop top or support bra.

8. And finally; during the first 1-12 weeks postpartum, is it recommended that women with implants book a consultation with their surgeon or their surgeon's nurse to check everything is ok with boobs/milk supply, etc? If so, when would you suggest is the best time to make this appointment? i.e. the first 4 weeks?

Not necessarily. Most women breastfeed their children with no issues and come back to see the surgeon when they're finished having kids for a 'Mummy makeover'. We say the 'door is always open'. But always recommend waiting at least 4 months from finishing breastfeeding before they come in. This allows the milk supply to be much less and we can properly assess the breast.

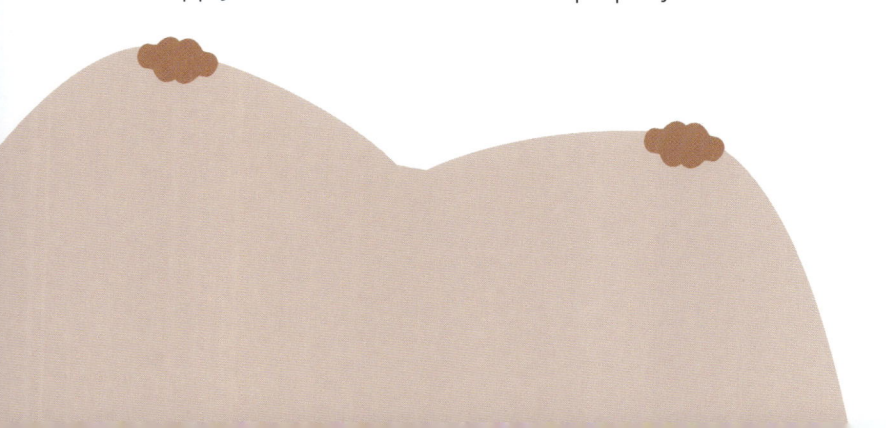

Again, if there are any issues (ongoing pain, swelling, etc.) this should be sooner and an ultrasound +/- MRI scan should be performed to check the implants/ surrounding breast tissue.

SUMMARY

Ah, boobs. Real ones, augmented ones, reduced ones, engorged ones, leaking ones, huge ones, tiny ones, painful ones, sick ones, lopsided ones, healing ones, recovered ones. They add a layer of complexity to the postpartum experience, don't they? They demand so much attention, they are as unpredictable as the newborn baby ... yet they provide nourishment ... and some great laughs over a glass of wine with a friend.

Cheers to you boobs.

quick hack

THE BREASTFEEDING BOX

When I was fed my bub during the first few months, I created a little basket that went everywhere with me, and I highly recommend the idea to all Mums. You never really know if you're going to be stuck feeding for 10, 30 or even 90 minutes at a time, so having the essentials in arms reach is a game changer. Where you go, the boob box follows.

◊ A Water Bottle … sip, sip, sip while feeding!

◊ Headphones … Podcasts were fab during feeds. My tops listens are Beyond The Bump, Shameless, Offline with Alison Rice, Life Uncut, Hello Bump, The Imperfects, Birth Baby & Beyond with Midwife Cath, The Remembering Project (Hamish & Andy), Gritty Pretty Radio, Interview with Andrew Denton, No Filter with Mia Freedman, ListenAble with Dylan Alcott and Angus O'Loughlin and Show + Tell Podcast

◊ Hair Elastics … there is nothing more irritating than hair in your face when breastfeeding

◊ Nipple Pads … when feeding with one boob, the other book is very likely to leak

◊ The Haakaa … to mitigate the above & save all the drips!

◊ Pen & Notebook … for all of the things you know you'll forget in 25 seconds time

◊ Stick on Eye Masks … why not give your eyes a little TLC while you have the time

◊ A Phone Charger … for obvious reasons

◊ A Flannel … for any leaks or spillage

◊ Snacks … muesli bars, raw balls, jelly beans, almonds

◊ Lip Balm & Facial Moisturiser… it's not uncommon to become dehydrated when you breastfeed which can lead to dry skin & lips

◊ Blue Light Glasses … for screen-time in the wee hours.

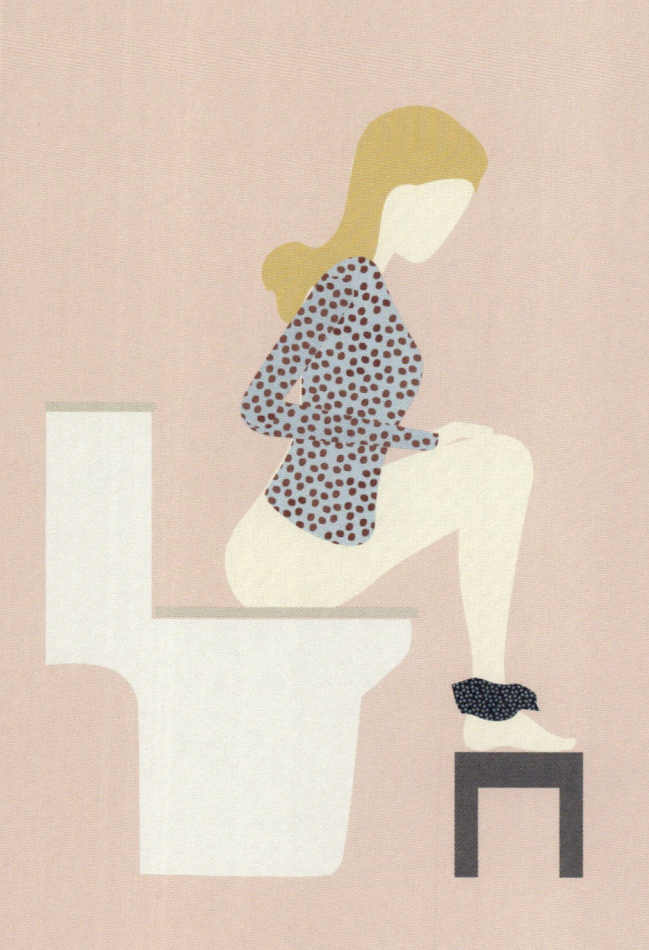

CHAPTER 4

Poo, Pads & Piddles

I think we can all comfortably admit that a common fear post-birth is doing your first poo … or the first few poos in the weeks following the birth. And fair enough! A whole human life (or potentially more), has just come out the front end & now the back end expects you to push something else out? This is a lot to ask of a person. Not to mention a person who probably has a very delicate wound in their abdomen or stitches between their vagina & their tooshie (and not the cute "cheeky" part of their tooshie… the hole).

Again, it is truly fair enough to fear doing a poo, so let's work out how to do this as comfortably and safely as possible whilst holding onto that thing called … eek what's that word again? Oh yes. Our dignity.

Firstly, it's not unusual if you're yet to feel the urge to go in the first few days. Constipation is common after giving birth which may make the thought of eventually "going" a little more daunting as the anxious thought "when will I go?" may circulate. Constipation is usually caused by dehydration (spanning from the loss of blood & fluids during birth), hormonal changes (for example increased progesterone levels), increased iron levels if you took supplements during pregnancy and/or just plain old fear around going. Your body might be doing its best to hold everything in as a defence mechanism, remembering that the last time you pushed something out of your body (your baby) it was a little painful. It's also worth noting that if you had a C-Section & have been more or less inactive during recovering this can certainly add fuel to the constipation fire as well.

Getting on top of constipation sooner rather than later is a good idea as you want to encourage your body to return to its regular functions. You also want to avoid Haemorrhoids. For anyone unsure about what a Haemorrhoids is, it's a swollen vessel around your rectum which can be either internal or external. They can be quite uncomfortable when you walk, sit or squat &

they can bleed when you go to the loo. While they're not super uncommon, Haemorrhoids ain't glamorous so avoiding them at all costs is a wise idea.

Below are some tips to help with constipation & prevent Haemorrhoids;

1. Drink plenty of water. Lots & lots of water especially if you're breastfeeding. A good idea is to buy yourself a big water bottle (1-2litres), before delivering to get organised. As you are so often sitting down with a baby glued to you in the early days, having a good water supply within arms reach is helpful.

2. Eat fresh! Eat lots of nutrient rich foods full of fibre goodness. Fruit, veggies, nuts & seeds, dried fruit, wholegrain bread … the lot!

3. When you feel the need to go, GO! Don't ignore the urge as it'll only exacerbate the issue.

4. Stool softeners can be very helpful, especially if you're battling a Hemorrhoid. Much like their name, they'll soften the poop making it easier & perhaps faster to pass. Easier & faster are two words we like after labour.

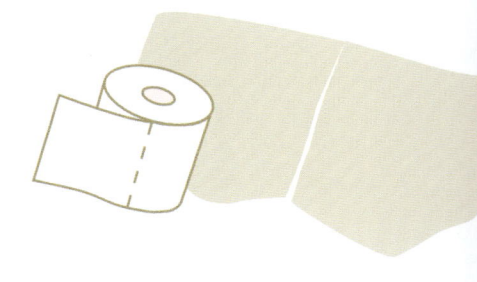

5. Look into probiotics. Some of the delicious yogurts on the market can do wonders in terms of creating movement. Yogurts with probiotic strains can very positively support the digestive system by maintaining a balanced gut microbiota. In a nutshell they can help to improve regularity.

You could also look into a probiotic supplement however it's highly recommended to check anything with your GP, midwife or maternal health nurse prior.

For those who look to laxatives when they're backed up, if you're breastfeeding (and/or pregnant) laxatives are not the best or the safest idea for several reasons. If you do want to go down the laxative route definitely check everything & anything with your your GP or the chemist first. You must stay away from self-prescribing when your mind, body, and bowel are tired and vulnerable. You've been through enough! You certainly don't need any other issues occurring.

Ok, so that covers what can help to keep you regular.

But when it comes to the actual act of sitting on the toilet & doing your business, let's now focus our attention here:

◊   **Hold Your Vagina:** This might sound a little ridiculous however it can offer a tremendous amount of comfort & support. As you push, with a clean hand position your palm over the vagina like a pad (use a maternity pad or a wad of toilet paper if you wish). You don't need to add a lot of pressure but if you feel like the pushing action will pop a stitch or push your vagina out of your body (which is a common postnatal fear), holding your vagina in place will ease your fears.

If you've had a C-Section you may like to hold a clean towel over your wound for the first few toilet visits. This will help to mitigate any unwanted abdominal pressure. The same goes for when you sneeze, cough & laugh.

- ◊ **Lean:** If you've had an Episiotomy or a tear, lean to the opposite side to where your stitches sit. If you don't know what side your stitches veer off to ask your midwife or the maternal health nurse when she next visits your home. Resting your body to one side by leaning on the wall, the toilet roll holder or even the toilet seat can offer great support.

- ◊ **Use The Door:** If it's available to you leave the toilet door open & lean forward to hold onto the door handle. Sitting down after birth can be quite uncomfortable, so removing some weight off your toosh may help.

- ◊ **Do The "Moo Poo":** Saying "MOO" while doing your business helps to increase intra-abdominal pressure & rectal pressure. This allows the stool to empty without too much strain on the pelvic floor and rectum.

- ◊ **Posture:** Using a footstool (see our lovely illustration), keep your knees higher than your hips & lean forwards as you make the "mooooo" sound. You'll feel your abdomen expand and some added pressure downwards in the rectum & anus which will assist with your bowel movement.

- ◊ **Don't Worry About Your Partner:** This bit is far easier said than done. It's very natural to feel a little shy about going to the loo, especially when you know you'll be in there a little longer than usual. If you are worried about what your partner might hear, smell, or whatever else - ask them to take the baby into another room & give you some much-deserved privacy. If it helps run the tap or play some music. If you let your pride defeat your poo you'll pay for it later.

- **Don't Over Do It:** If you're pushing with no relief it's probably best to stop trying. You need to think about your pelvic floor here. It's tired & weak and it doesn't need anything upsetting its best efforts to recover. Up the fluids, try & go for a slow walk and load up on fibre rich food. Think prunes, fresh Medjool dates, fruit toast, chia pods, fresh salads and leafy greens. Maybe even throw in a few glasses of Metamucil during the day.

Pooping is a part of life. It's not the most pleasant part of life ... but a crucial part nonetheless. If you're someone who tends to hold angst, worry, fear, or loads of emotion in your belly, this may cause your bowel to explode or freeze. Either outcome is not ideal so checking in with your poops post-birth is always a good habit.

HYGIENE

Women who have had stitches due to an Episiotomy or a tear will need to be super vigilant about keeping their wounds clean. This means being very careful when wiping.

Have a read over the below as keeping clean & fresh is paramount.

- Keep thoroughly washing your hands before & after dealing with the downstairs region.
- Ladies, like you're taught when you are toilet trained; Front To Back.
- Similar to after having a spray tan ... follow the "gentle pat dry," advice.

- ◊ If it adds comfort, keep unscented wet wipes in the bathroom. Gently use them to "pat dry" or clean yourself post poo instead of dry toilet paper.

- ◊ After doing a poop if you can hop straight into a warm shower and rinse off, do it! If you need to do this more than once a day, so be it. Enjoy the peaceful shower time and let your partner, family member or a friend care for the bubba for 5-10 minutes. Whilst in the shower it's advisable to avoid soap as it may sting & it's not required.

- ◊ Change your maternity pads* every 2-4hours.

- ◊ Keep your underwear fresh, especially if you're using maternity pads. A clean pair of undies is like brushing your teeth. Instant fresh feels!

*A quick note on maternity pads. If you're currently using normal pads but for a heavy flow or for nighttime wear, stick to maternity pads as they are by far the best solution. Despite looking so similar, maternity pads are carefully designed for this tender part of life. Comfort and hygiene are everything. Maternity pads are longer, more adsorbent and most importantly they're designed without the plastic mesh which may stick to your stitches or irritate your wound.

On the topic of hygiene … before we close the PPP chapter, let's chat a little more about pads.

DISPOSAL OF MATERNITY PADS

Ok, so these things are like nappies … let's call a spade a spade … and if you're changing them every 4 hours, that's 6-12 ginormous pads to dispose of every single day. This may sound like a sweeping generalisation however women can be very shy about sanitary products, especially used sanitary products. When you buy them they're super cute and colourful but when the wrapper come off it's time to get them out of sight.

I hope this doesn't sound too vulgar (but it's true) used maternity pads are likely to have an odour. It'd be cruel to feel embarrassed if this is true in your case, so go easy. It's beyond natural! You've just had a baby, your world is spinning & your body is exceptionally vulnerable and probably incredibly uncomfortable as well. Take a breath, so many other women are feeling your feels.

Here are some quick tips on the subject to bright you lightness & ease;

- Buy a bin with a lid & keep it next to your toilet or very close to your toilet (i.e. in the same room). Make sure the bin is lined with a disposable bag so you can untie & re-tie it every time you dispose of a pad. If you don't have a bin send your partner off to Kmart, Big W, Officeworks, Coles, Ikea, Target or Woolies.

- When you remove a pad from your underwear, fold it up & wrap it in toilet paper before you place it in the bin bag. Not essential but more hygienic and considerate to the people living with you.

- Keep your maternity pads and/or your sanitary disposal bags next to the toilet. It might also be a good idea to keep a pack of unscented baby wipes next to the toilet as well (scented wipes may sting your wound) just in case they offer you a more comfortable solution to toilet paper. If it helps buy a cute box or a basket for all of these cute things to live in.

◊ There is a lot to do with a brand new baby in the house, but changing this bin bag daily is a good habit to get into. Keeping things fresh is nice.

It can feel humiliating when you're changing a boat-sized maternity pad every 2-4 hours. It can feel embarrassing when you have an accident and need to change your underwear or your entire outfit more than once daily. It can feel mortifying and yucky when you forget to grab a new pad & have to roll up a wad of toilet paper as a short-term solution.

For every nappy change it feels like there's a pad change. For every accident of the babies there may be an accident of your own. A wee, a bleed, a boob leak. It can feel exhausting, unclean, and immensely undignified when you realise that you need just as much assistance downstairs as your newborn baby.

Yep, it absolutely can. Wearing two pairs of underwear for the first few weeks or months might offer a little comfort and a lot of reassurance regarding the fear of leaking. Black, firm underwear is a good idea as things will feel well supported and safe. Those lacy g's and Brazilian cuts in your drawer? They can take a hike for a little while.

Rest assured that every single woman who has gone through this postpartum patch of time before you has shared these common worries and mourned for their pre-baby sense of femininity, predictability & self-control. No one likes to have an accident. This phase will pass.

Shall we now talk about the final P in the chapter, PIDDLES? Why not!

WEE

Pre-baby, I bet so many women reading this (like myself), looked at the Tena incontinence pads on the shelves at the supermarket & thought to themselves, "How hard is it not to wee unless you're on the toilet?"

Well since having a baby it turns out weeing is quite an art form. It's not the wee, it's the holding it in part that can be tough. Anyone else running the shower or getting to the front door & to then have to sprint to the bathroom to relieve your bladder?

The bladder is similar to a balloon. When it's full with urine it's held firmly in place by the surrounding pelvic floor muscles. As we've mentioned a few times, when women are pregnant the release of the Relaxin hormone can soften your muscles, making them more elastic and potentially a little weaker than usual. In some cases a lot weaker than usual. When the body makes an unexpected movement i.e. a laugh, a cough, a jump, or a sneeze - the bladder may lack the strength to squeeze tightly enough to hold in the urine. This causes the urine to sneak through the urethra … or in other words this causes you to suddenly wee yourself. You might not drench your undies but you'll feel damp and uncomfortable.

Adding to this when women deliver vaginally as the baby comes down the birth canal the pelvic floor stretches and it may remain stretched for some time. Women may suffer varying degrees of postpartum bladder incontinence for a few weeks or months. Some women may unfortunately never fully recover their pre-baby pelvic floor stretch. To avoid being in the latter group have a read below;

Ways To Prevent Incontinence

- Practice your Kegal exercises daily. Not weekly or monthly or annually … daily.

- ◊ Try and retrain your bladder in the days, weeks & months that follow your birth. When you need to do a wee hold on for a little longer allowing your bladder to fill.

- ◊ Similar to above try and avoid going to the loo every time you feel a faint urge to wee. Side Note; I can appreciate this is VERY hard. If I had a dollar for every time I woke up during the night and listened to this internal discussion;

"Do I need to pee? Nah I'll be ok. NO GET UP, YOU NEED TO PEE! Yeah but … what if I just wait until I'm really busting? You are REALLY busting NOW. No I'm not - you're being a drama queen."

2 minutes later.

"Just go now so you can go back to sleep before the baby cries. But the walk to the bathroom will wake me up? YOU ARE AWAKE NOW! And do you know what's keeping you awake? This conversation!!! I think it'll be fine, I only drank about 3 sips… no. Maybe about 7 sips of water? What's 7 sips, like half a glass? Is that a lot in terms of the size of my bladder? JUST GO!…. Fine. but if I wake the baby or if no wee comes out, I'll be super pissed."

- ◊ Maintain a healthy weight for your height and build. Your pelvic floor doesn't want to support any more weight than it needs to right now. Doing your very best to keep on top of your general wellbeing needs to be a priority. Eat good food (plenty of fresh fruits & vegetables), limit your alcohol intake, and avoid smoking.

- ◊ Visit a trusted women's health physio who will help to improve your bladder control in a personalised way. Guided feedback is of so much value.

That should cover poo, pads & piddle for now? Even though they're not the frilliest of subjects, let's be thankful we didn't have to add a fourth P into the mix. **PERIODS**.

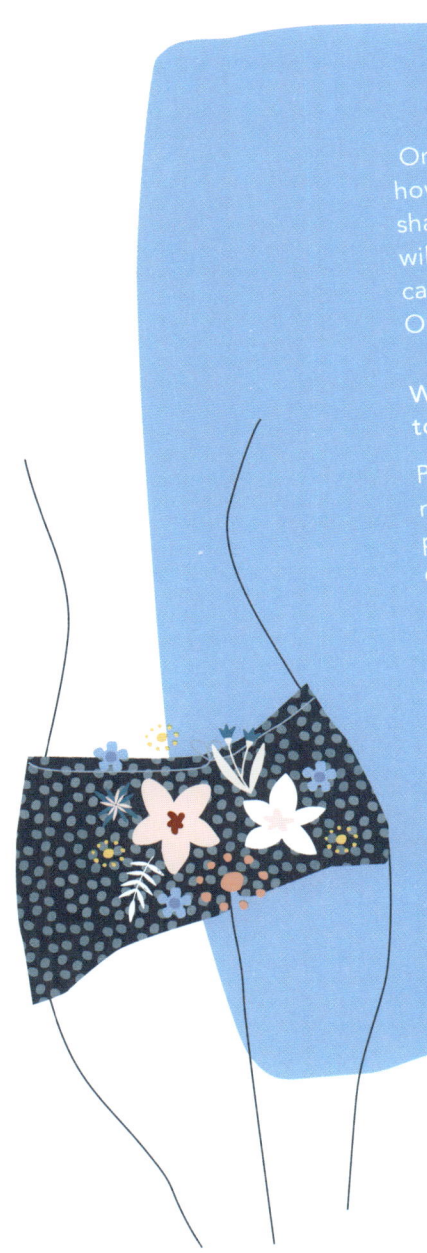

On the topic of periods however, a common curiosity shared by new Mums is when will it return? Once again, let's call on our midwife Sophie Outwaite for this one...

When might women expect to get their period back?

Prolactin, the hormone responsible for breast milk production, also suppresses ovulation. Therefore, for women who exclusively breastfeed it is normal not to menstruate for six months or longer. Many women don't menstruate at all until they stop breastfeeding altogether. Women who don't breastfeed usually find their menstrual cycle returns to normal between four to eight weeks following childbirth

Letters to myself...

Dear me,

I'm aware that my shorts are filthy. I think I sat on my croissant. Now come to think of it, where is that croissant? I am starving. And my apple? Did I eat that? Or was it a banana they bought me? Where is the banana? x

CHAPTER 5

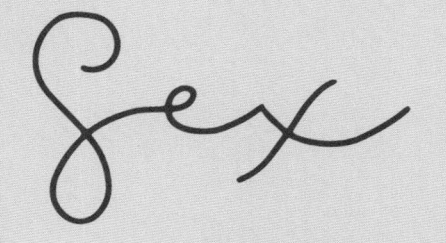

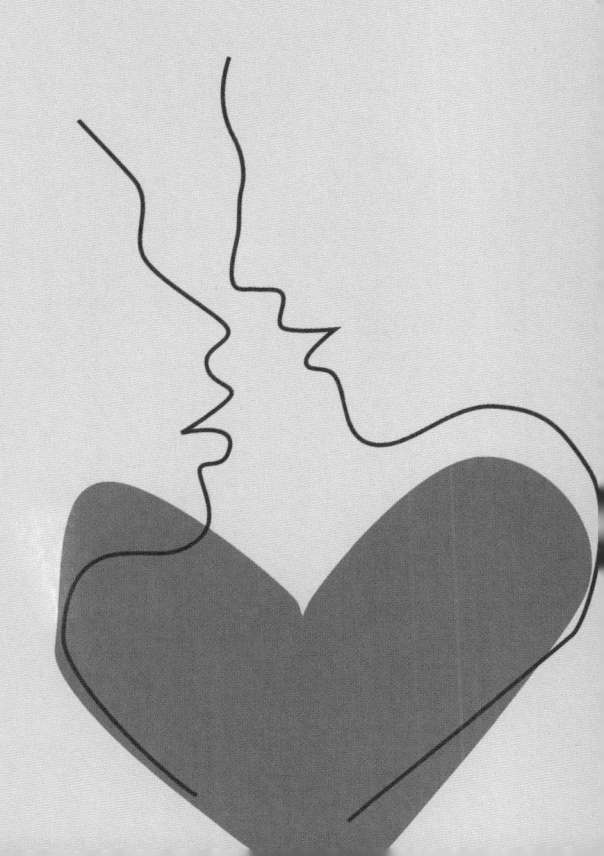

Sex

P 96   AFTERWARDS

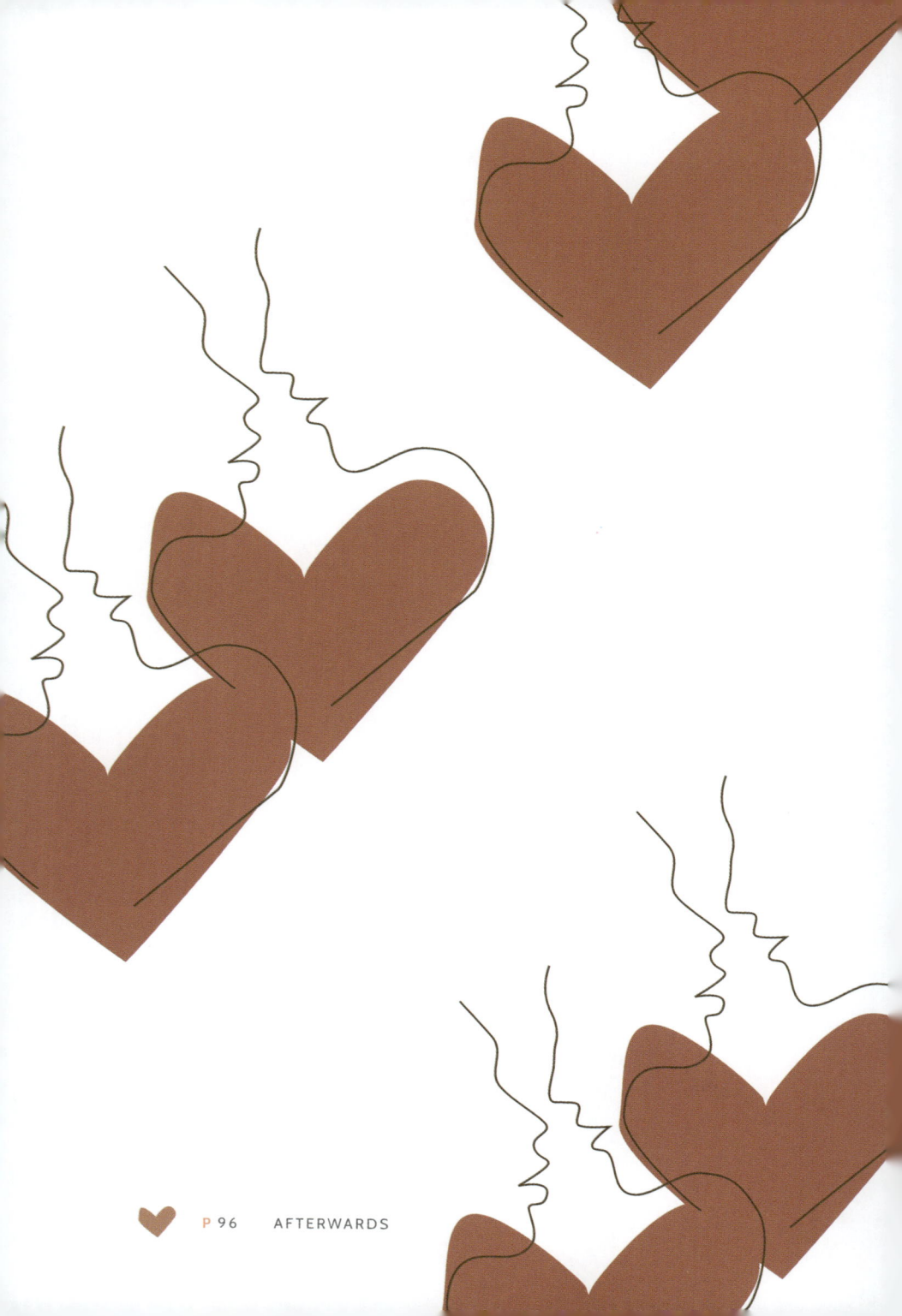

Sex is a funny postpartum subject. An intense one. A BIG one. A scary one! Sex is the exact thing that landed us in the puddle of postpartum water in the first place so why on earth would women voluntarily jump back in? Why is the major question. When is another … and HOW? The how element deserves some careful unpacking as having a shag after you birth your bub can be undeniably daunting.

In many ways it shares similarities to the common story involving a dog getting jammed between a closing door as a puppy. The dog never forgets the terror associated with that moment & forever seems to fear the mere sight of a doorway.

Whilst you're imagining the above replace the door with a doodle. Oh, and while you're at it replace the puppy with a vulnerable, emotional & tired new Mum.

YIKES.

Ya.

So while that is an overly negative way to think about sex we should admit & acknowledge that sex is a huge part of our lives, our relationships, and the closeness of our connections. Sex should be enjoyable, fun and exciting! If you want to crave it again or eventually add to your brood, then it's critical to work up the courage to get through that metaphorical doorway again. We need to trust that it won't harshly slam shut on our backside but instead lead us into a space where we can relax & indulge.

Before moving forward it's important to recognise that the fear or the hesitation you may be struggling with is totally valid. I'm sure a snippet of PTSD sneaks into the minds of most women when they think about returning to sex for the first time after having their baby … and perhaps even the 2nd time, the 10th time … the 50th time!

To avoid adding to any angst let's very gently break it down and look into the why's, the what's, and the how's. To help us do so the Director of the Australian Institute of Sexology and Sexual Medicine & ESSM EFS Certified Psycho-Sexologist, Chantelle Otten (@chantelle_otten_sexologist), has very kindly shared her highly demanded time & advice with everyone who is reading this.

Chantelle is passionate about sex & relationships and is devoted to making sure that women exude pride & confidence in both their beautiful body & their sexuality. Her tips & tricks are there to encourage a positive relationship with sex whilst always prioritising a woman's choice, her health, and of course, her safety. As she poignantly quotes below during our interview ' the only person responsible for your pleasure is you," … Chantelle certainly offers an abundance of wise & considerate guidance.

Ok enough from me. Let's talk to this wonderful powerhouse!

1. It's not uncommon for partners to watch the birth of their baby & therefore see everything. This may cause extreme insecurities for women & cause them to feel as though they won't be as attractive again to their partners. Is there a way you'd suggest they tackle this fear?

Childbirth no matter what method of delivery has a significant impact on the female body. Understanding that these feelings are completely normal and positively approaching insecurities can help to repair the relationship with your body from the late stages of pregnancy into the postpartum period. Celebrate and thank your body for all it has done for you; it has grown and birthed a human! Practice self-compassion, be kind to yourself and make time for the little things that make you feel good about yourself such as a bath or wearing a beautiful maternity bra. Additionally, facilitate an open dialogue with your partner about how you're feeling and any insecurities, worries, or concerns. The chances are that they are amazed and in awe of what your body is capable of.

2. Physical pain is a real factor when it comes to sex post-birth. Whether women have a c-section or vaginal birth, their bodies go through some extreme measures. If it hurts, do you suggest stopping cold turkey? Is pain sign of an issue?

There can be many different reasons for postpartum sexual pain such as lack of vaginal lubrication, trauma to the vagina, prolapse, or tightness in the pelvic floor. Pain can act as an indicator that something else is going on or it can act as a protective mechanism to prevent the body from experiencing any further trauma. If women are experiencing sexual pain I recommend stopping all forms of vaginal penetration. This will allow you to feel safe knowing that physical touch doesn't have to end in vaginal penetration whilst still receiving touch and connection that is often desired through sex.

Sex should never be painful. Seek help from a medical practitioner such as an OB/GYN or a pelvic floor physiotherapist if you are experiencing sexual pain.

3. Despite potential pain, some women may crave sex earlier than the loosely suggested 6 week period. What are some tactics to safely ease back into it?

The 6-week guideline exists to allow the vagina and abdomen to sufficiently heal following birth. For those who want to engage in sexual penetration before the recommended 6-week point, it is essential to get clearance from your OB/GYN. However, that is not to say that you can't enjoy other items on the sexual menu such as masturbation, oral sex, or even an erotic massage. Listening to the body in this instance is paramount. And don't forget, lube - lots and lots of lube.

QUICK INTERRUPTION HERE! To add to Chantelle's expert advice, our midwife Sophie Outhwaite shares her comments on the 6-week timeframe just to reiterate why this particular timeframe is so commonly advised.

Soph, when is it safe to return to sex post baby?

Irrespective of how you gave birth, most doctors will advise you wait at least 6 weeks post-delivery. By this time you've probably attended your postnatal 6 week check with your GP, your lochia should have stopped and unless you had postnatal complications, your episiotomy, lacerations or grazes (if you had any) should have healed.

4. Ok. The boobs. They probably don't match, they might be engorged, sore, leaky & exceptionally sensitive ... & not in a good way! For Mummas who are self-conscious about how their boobs may look during sex, what would perhaps be some more "flattering" positions? The point here isn't vanity - it's allowing women to feel sexy in their own skin!

Each experience is individual so it is important to experiment to find a position that YOU feel most comfortable in. That being said positions that take the pressure off the breasts such as lying on the back or the side (with their partner behind them) may not only look more flattering but also help with any leaking that may occur. Additionally, wearing beautiful lingerie can help to cover the areas that make women feel self-conscious whilst still feeling sexy.

5. For severely sleep-deprived women, suffering from engorgement or sore nipples & enduring heavy night sweats ... yet all the while feeling guilty that they're unable to find their mojo for their partners' sake ... what would you tell these women?

Couples are faced with extreme change in a short amount of time and it is entirely normal to experience a downward shift in libido during the postpartum period. Be kind to yourself and communicate with your partner how you are feeling. If penetration is off the table and desire seems like a foreign term perhaps focus on intimate touches such as a hug, a kiss, or holding hands to foster that emotional connection and intimacy. Remember that the newborn phase is only temporary and your libido will eventually return.

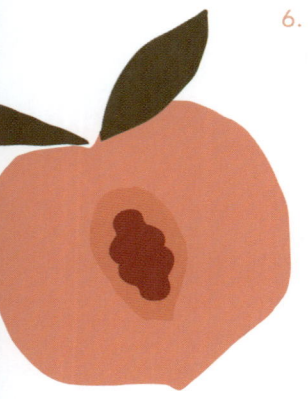

6. Vaginismus is no joke! Can you explain this & perhaps offer some solutions to eradicate the mental hurdles it creates?

Vaginismus is the involuntary tightening of the pelvic floor muscles surrounding the vagina making penetration incredibly painful or impossible. It can feel like burning, tearing or razor blade-like sensations inside and around the entrance of the vagina. The reasons that vaginismus can occur in the postpartum period can vary; perhaps you have experienced traumatic birth or the first time you had sex was particularly painful. Your body is subconsciously serving to protect itself from further pain. Vaginismus can have a substantial emotional impact on self-esteem, sexual/relationship satisfaction and quality of life. If you feel like you might have vaginismus please get help immediately! It is one of the most treatable conditions. A multi-disciplinary approach to treatment is key so seeking help from a sexologist as well as a pelvic floor physiotherapist will address the physical as well as psychological hurdles that may be occurring.

7. Let's get down & dirty. Could you recommend a few specific positions for new Mums who are ready to get goin'! Keeping in mind they probably need to be gentle to aid their recovery?

◊ Missionary Position: lying down helps to relax the pelvic floor muscles and legs - communication is essential to discern the speed and pressure that is comfortable.

◊ Cowgirl/Reverse Cowgirl Position: being on top allows complete control of the depth of penetration and pace.

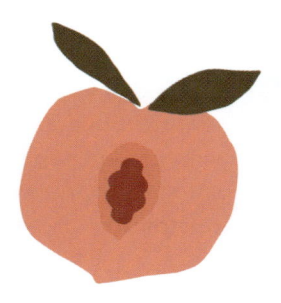

◊ Spooning Position: lying on the side to take the pressure off the body and to increase intimate touch. Allows for clitoral stimulation and also helps women to feel more comfortable if they are self-conscious about their body.

8. Some women feel as though with the role of motherhood, comes the loss of their sex appeal, femininity & sense of self-worth. How do women rebuild a healthy relationship with their bodies?

Becoming a mother can have a significant impact on identity and sense of self, and for the first few weeks of motherhood the focus is primarily on keeping your newborn alive. Your body and perception of who you are has likely changed and that is ok. There is a societal perception that motherhood and sexual being do not co-exist. However, it is the confidence in being able to separate caring for a child and prioritising your relationship and pleasure that work to integrate the two. Focusing on necessary self-care such as making time for a shower and wearing things that make you feel beautiful can help reclaim that sense of identity. Prioritise your partner and quality time together to reinforce that your relationship is vital to who you are. It may take some time to find your feet, and if you are struggling, reaching out to a sexologist can help reclaim that sense of self-worth.

9. A rainbow of hormones floods the body after birth. What hormones can trigger sexual feelings? And how can they be harnessed positively?

Within 4-6 weeks postpartum estrogen and progesterone levels plummet leading to decreased sexual desire and a natural reduction in vaginal lubrication. This, in conjunction with prolactin (if nursing), also suppresses libido. For women who are not nursing prolactin stabilises around 4-6 weeks postpartum. Even after hormonal levels have stabilised it is normal to experience lower libido than prior to pregnancy due to contextual factors such as fatigue, feeling self-conscious in your changing body and the potential diagnosis of post-natal depression or anxiety. If you think that your hormones may still be out of whack don't hesitate to get this checked out by your doctor. Managing the biological side (hormones) along with the psychological side (your context around you that is leading to low libido) can help to foster sexual desire.

10. Dryness downstairs whilst breastfeeding is very common. Why does the vagina become so dry & how can women overcome the issue to ensure they enjoy sex?

Breastfeeding has a significant impact on sexual functioning one that isn't spoken about enough. One of the main consequences of breastfeeding is vaginal dryness caused by the hormone prolactin. Prolactin also inhibits ovulation affecting the menstrual cycle and the natural fluctuations in estrogen and progesterone thereby negatively impacting libido. This is to allow the mother to focus on her baby rather than future procreation. Moreover a significant lack of sleep and constantly caring for a newborn is not conducive to arousal and vaginal lubrication. During the postpartum phase lube is your best friend. Opt for one that is water-based and pH balanced so it does not cause further irritation.

11. A couple of wines to get back on the horse ... something you'd suggest?

This is a personal preference. Given the likelihood that new mothers may be nursing consider the impact that alcohol can have on breastfeeding. The premise behind the 'glass of wine' advice is that it helps you to relax; however, research shows that more than two glasses of wine can negatively impact on sexual functioning. Rather than reaching for the wines explore other ways of relieving stress and anxiety to get you in the mood such as running a warm bath or shower with your partner, candles or low lighting, a sexy playlist, and being intimate with your partner in ways that don't necessarily involve vaginal penetration.

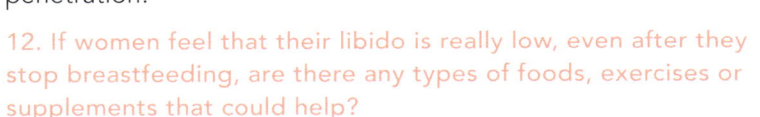

12. If women feel that their libido is really low, even after they stop breastfeeding, are there any types of foods, exercises or supplements that could help?

From a biological perspective it is important to have hormones tested either by a doctor or a naturopath to see if they are within a normal range. A medical practitioner would then guide treatment for this to rebalance hormones as this can have a significant impact on energy and libido.

From a psychological perspective explore the contextual factors that could be contributing to low libido such as feelings of anxiety, sleep deprivation, low body image etc. Working with a sexologist during the postpartum period can be beneficial for women and their partners in managing expectations around desire and sex.

13. If women feel the need to fake pleasure or orgasms, purely for the enjoyment of their partners post-baby … what is your advice?

Perhaps ask yourself why you feel the need to fake pleasure and orgasms with your partner. It is completely normal that your experience of pleasure has probably changed and this could mean that you may need to spend some time relearning what feels good in your body. A great place to start is through masturbation. Explore pleasure in your body, be open and curious, and experiment with how and where you like to be touched. If you know what gives you pleasure this will make it a lot easier communicating this to your partner. Remember, the only person responsible for your pleasure is you.

...

I hope that within these pages you've been able to find pockets of inspired ideas which you can welcome between your sheets. Don't rush it or force it & if there is pain refrain from moving forward. Pain is your body's way of telling you that it is not ready or something isn't quite right. Be kind to yourself & remove all pressure!

Postpartum life aside Chantelle is a woman I'd highly suggest following on social media. Her content, advice and words are intelligent, generous, zealous, electric & real. She not only encourages a pure relationship with your body & sex but she teaches the world how to unlock the rich treasure hidden inside each & every individual.

Back to the first shag post-birth, when you decide that it's your time to go back & give sex a go, as you roll around on the bed like a nervous teenager, don't sweat it if you cry in fear or fumble in an awkward moment. If you blush, cringe, clench or slap your partner away with accidental or spontaneous force … there will be no love lost. Allow time to be your friend.

Another fun & fabulous podcast to tune into is **Birth, Baby & Beyond; Sex After Birth** - Is It Fun? (available on Podcast One). This particular podcast features the infamous Midwife Cath plus two other exceptionally knowledgeable, experienced, and wonderfully humorous women Brooke Carrigan and Dr. Sue Hiscock. Birth, Baby & Beyond is a refreshing & light listen that so honestly breakdowns EVERYTHING you are thinking about this topic. Pop your Air Pods in and enjoy the warmth this trio offers.

Like we said in the first chapter, perhaps it's best to do yourself a favour and roll over to remind old mate to not be a fool & cover his tool! In other, slightly more ladylike terms, find a method of contraception that suits your body & mental health and ... well use it. You can begin your quest to breed a tribe of mini people when you've caught up on sleep & once again experienced wearing underwear that isn't stuffed with pads the size of The Titanic & icepacks.

quick hack

WHILE YOU FEED, YOUR PARTNER CAN …

◊ Vacuum the floors or wipe up the milk drips on the floor

◊ Hang or fold the washing

◊ Make sure that your water bottle & the remote control are always within reach

◊ Sterilise the baby bottles

◊ Sort out that chaotic cupboard that's been keeping you up at night

◊ Do their best to breathe at a pitch or tempo that is not annoying or infuriating

◊ Book in a Baby First Aid Course

◊ Cook dinners or pop to the shops

◊ Read you the newspaper or funny memes

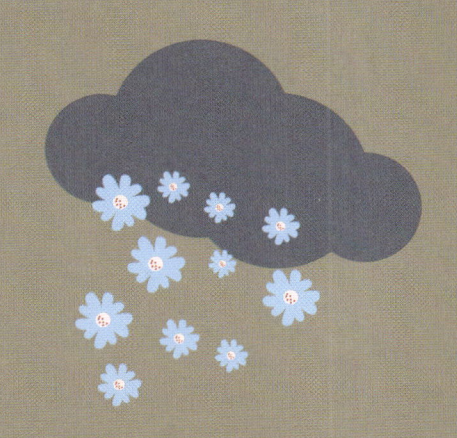

◊ Try & avoid asking questions that are unnecessary and that have obvious answers anyway. For example, Do you mind if I go to the pub tonight? May I eat the last Banjo Carob Bear? Mind if we turn the cricket on? Regarding the latter, should your partner need a friendly hint, I'd say an alternative phrasing might be … Do you mind if I check the cricket score?

◊ Sit with you & keep you company because it's nice to be near someone you adore

◊ Fill a blank spot in your mind. For example, before "…the dish ran away with the spoon", what was it that the dog did again?

◊ Remind you that you're doing a good job. Even if the baby is crying or not having a bar of the latch, you are doing A Good Job.

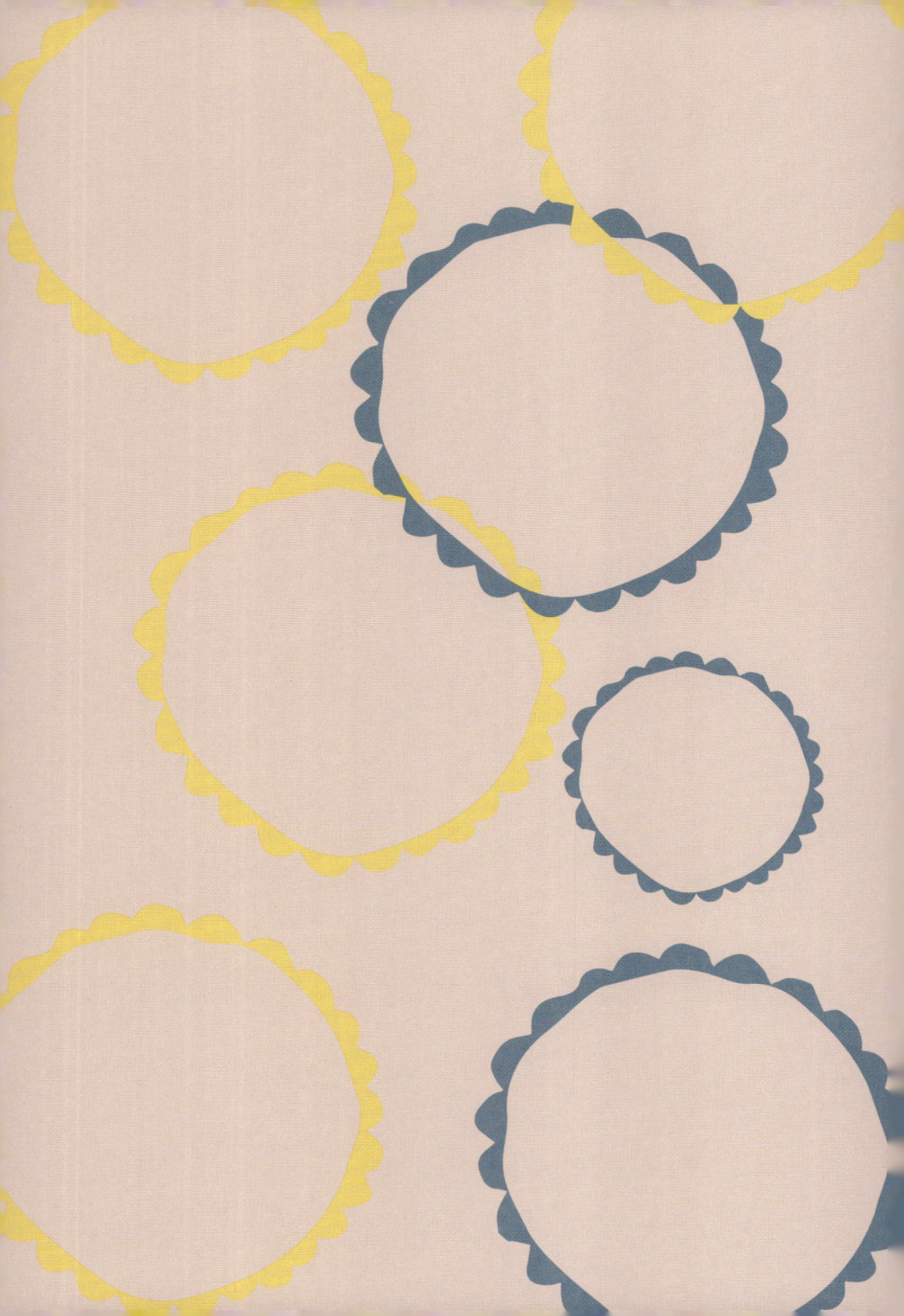

CHAPTER 6

Postpartum & The Big C

P 112   AFTERWARDS

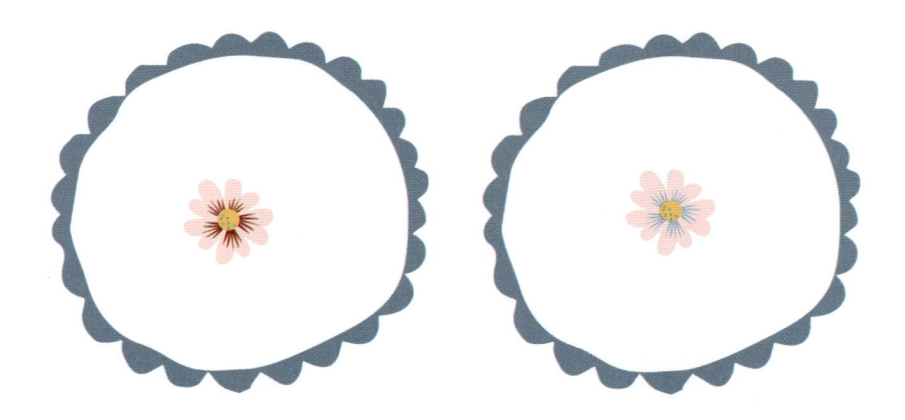

It is true that post birth new Mums deal with fractured sleep, odd worries, cramps & aches around their coccyx, hips & their back. It is true that some new Mums go through waves of blue where they cry tears of panic or feel an unpredictable, deep sadness if postpartum depression or anxiety finds a way into their heart. Like this isn't enough?

But for some there is more to handle, much more. For some there is breast cancer. A cruel, dispassionate disease that joylessly snuggles bodies & bones that should only ever house pleasure & budding life. And so unfortunately, some of those to be cornered by cancer are new, beautiful young mothers who deserve everything but this viscous diagnosis.

According the Breast Cancer Network Australia (BCNA), in 2021, an estimated 20,825 Australians will be diagnosed with breast cancer. That is 1 in every 7 Australian woman. Too many.

Raising awareness and encouraging all women of all ages & at different points of life, to be super vigilant when it comes to checking their breasts and familiarising themselves with any changes to their look & feel, is a critical message to spread. While cancer does not discriminate, it may offer its unlucky host a small clue alluding to their sheepish intention… "I'm coming" or worst yet, "I'm here, all guns blazing."

Below is an interview with the brave & wonderfully inspirational Emily Halberg. A 31 year old picture of health who just 3 months after welcoming her gorgeous baby boy Finn into the world, was diagnosed with breast cancer. Please read this interview & remind yourself just how radically life can turn when you least expect it and when you least deserve it. This isn't to evoke fear or distress … this is to encourage awareness and celebrate action, bravery and truth.

Within the coming pages, Em bravely tells us the story of her diagnosis, her treatment and her emotional journey as she navigates her way through cancer while simultaneously transitioning into her first year as a mother (and a bloody amazing one at that!!). I can't thank her enough for sharing such a personal chapter of her life. Em ignites what we all should strive for - gratitude, selflessness & pure perspective.

1. Can you tell us a little about the journey to your diagnosis?

A little about me at the time of diagnosis. I'm 31 years old, healthy as a clam (regarding diet/weight/lifestyle), and I have been blessed with a beautiful 3 month old boy, Finn. One day whilst expressing I felt a small lump in my right breast, on the cusp of where my breast meets my underarm, and thought perhaps a blocked milk duct. I had heard before that lumpy breasts are common in 'breastfeeding Mums'.

A week later I saw my GP and mentioned the lump in a fly away comment. She suggested an ultrasound and if required, a biopsy, to be sure it wasn't anything nasty. The following week I had the ultrasound, with feedback that there is a 1% chance it would be cancerous due to its unusually perfect circular shape. I took the gamble none the less and booked for the biopsy the soonest availability. At the biopsy I was told I've have results back from the biopsy via my GP within 5 days. Scarily I heard from my GP within 18 hours of the biopsy, asking for an urgent appointment with myself and my husband, Nev, leaving Finn at home. My heart sank. At the GP we were told I had breast cancer and they were unsure how far it had progressed. And due to the unusual shape, they couldn't guarantee it hadn't spread. It was likely stage 3 based on its size alone, and I couldn't be certain I'd see my Finn's first birthday.

The following day I was in and out of appointments checking the rest of my body. All I could think about was Finn and that no matter what, I had to do everything in my power to be there for him and Nev.

We were so lucky. The results returned that afternoon advising it was limited to the breast only. It was a 4.5cm tumour and I needed to start chemo the following week. That evening my husband and I went to our local restaurant to celebrate that my cancer was unlikely terminal, it was the best news of my life. We had a bottle of excellent chardonnay and toasted to life.

2. In terms of breastfeeding & caring for your baby, how does the treatment change your day-to-day?

Sadly my breastfeeding and expressing had to stop as soon as I commenced chemo. I expressed up until my first round of chemo, then took tablets to expedite drying up my milk supply. As Finn was 3 months old, my milk was well established, so stopping my supply was another task I had to manage. I had to balance expressing to dump to mitigate engorgement but not express too much and build my supply. Expressing was painful as a side effect of chemo is skin sensitivity, so pulling my sensitive nipples through a flange to then dump the milk was the absolute definition of no-fun-at-all.

In some ways I felt so guilty that I had to stop providing breastmilk for Finn, but I would feel more guilty for declining chemo or delaying chemo and potentially not being there for Finn in his future. Finn's transition to formula was excellent. He was used to a bottle already so latching onto the teat & feeling familiar with the silicone was no issue. We had 2 days of unusual (green) nappies when we went cold turkey to formula, but otherwise no change in demeanour, attitude, sleep or weight.

3. Experiencing such a harrowing ordeal so soon after the arrival of your first beautiful baby seems unimaginably unfair. What encourages your spirited nature and your motivation to tackle this illness with so much heart?

It was such shocking news to be diagnosed with breast cancer, with no family history or 'reason' why I could be at risk of having it. But when we heard the news, that it was treatable, I felt euphoric. The only thing that mattered was being there for my family. Soon after my diagnosis I heard one in eight women get breast cancer in their lives. Sure, most of these women are in their later years of life, but I thought, if me having breast cancer has spared my seven closest friends and family from having it, heck I'd take it again.

4. For the many people around you who so desperately want to help, what means the most/helps the most?

Messages from friends saying 'I've booked in to get a breast check," Wow, that really meant so much. If my story and experience could prevent someone from going through this, then that is the greatest gift I could receive. I also really appreciated people privately reaching out, or stopping me on the street and giving me a hug saying, 'I'm so sorry to hear what you're going through, that's awful'. Thank you for not ignoring it, or avoiding the awkward conversation. Good on you, friend.

Everyone has been so generous in their capacity. We have received so many beautiful hampers, flowers, meal deliveries, referrals to exceptional doctors, vouchers, fragrance free beauty products etc, all so generous. The thought that has gone into these gifts has been overwhelmingly kind.

5. In moments of weakness and exhaustion, how do you find comfort? Or is it more about reaching deep and finding ways to sit with the discomfort, knowing (or hoping), a wave of relief will come eventually?

Recognition that this experience is not a sprint, it's a marathon.

Although the marathon feels like forever, the chapters are short, and temporary. Bone soreness is temporary, nausea is temporary, 16 weeks of chemo is temporary, it's for my longer term survival

My need to survive isn't for my benefit me anymore, it's about being there for my family.

6. Your message to other women?

Check your boobies, men and women!

If there is something on your mind, niggling you in the back of your brain and you think 'that just doesn't feel right', get a test done. Sending a beautiful bunch of flowers to a friend with cancer costs the same as getting your breasts/body checked, and as the friend with cancer, I know which option I would prefer you spend your money on. I want to spread awareness that breast cancer isn't limited to women in their 40's when we're only 'required' to get mammograms, no one is exempt from cancer.

At first I felt embarrassed walking around my local shops with no head hair, eye brows and thinning lashes, but that is the reality of cancer, why put on a hat or wig and pretend everything is perfect? We are the generation of spreading awareness and our stories and although I'm mortified that my ears stick out, I think Finn will grow up hearing he had a strong, resilient Mumma, and I hope he'd be proud of me. Through this journey haven't felt sorry for myself. I haven't thought 'Why me', really, why not me? I'm a person, there is a chance I would develop cancer, I just drew the short straw getting it at 31 years old. I haven't been told how I developed breast cancer, potentially the tumour has been sitting dormant for years, and I only just felt it because I was expressing, or maybe it was due to a spike in hormones through pregnancy that brought it on, but I wouldn't change my journey to date, so I am embracing it, treating it as a 'health speed bump' in an otherwise very long (hopefully) and happy life.

7. Your message to yourself?

The priority must be on survival and being there for my family. It can't be weight management, keeping up with the social scene, exercising to look good in bathers, it just has to be on survival, and anything else I can muster is a bonus. Be kind to your calendar and carve out the days you know you'll feel terrible and just focus on being there for Finn.

Losing your hair is terrible - it's a choice which is taken away from you when it's been a choice you've had your whole life. It makes a very personal health experience, public. But losing your hair doesn't change who you are, it actually just adds to your character.

It's okay my clothes don't fit, you're injecting your body with hours of toxic infusions fortnightly, of course you're going to feel and look different!

Spend time with the people who give you energy, who ask you are going but don't dwell on it. Yes, I've got cancer, it's not my full identity. I'm also a mother, a wife, a daughter, a sister, and a friend. I am more than a tumour in my breast.

Finn Born: 3 August 2020
Diagnosis: 5 November 2020
Chemotherapy: 20 November 2020 - 1 March 2021 (fortnightly)
Surgery Date: 23 March 2021
Radiation: Mid April to End of May 2021

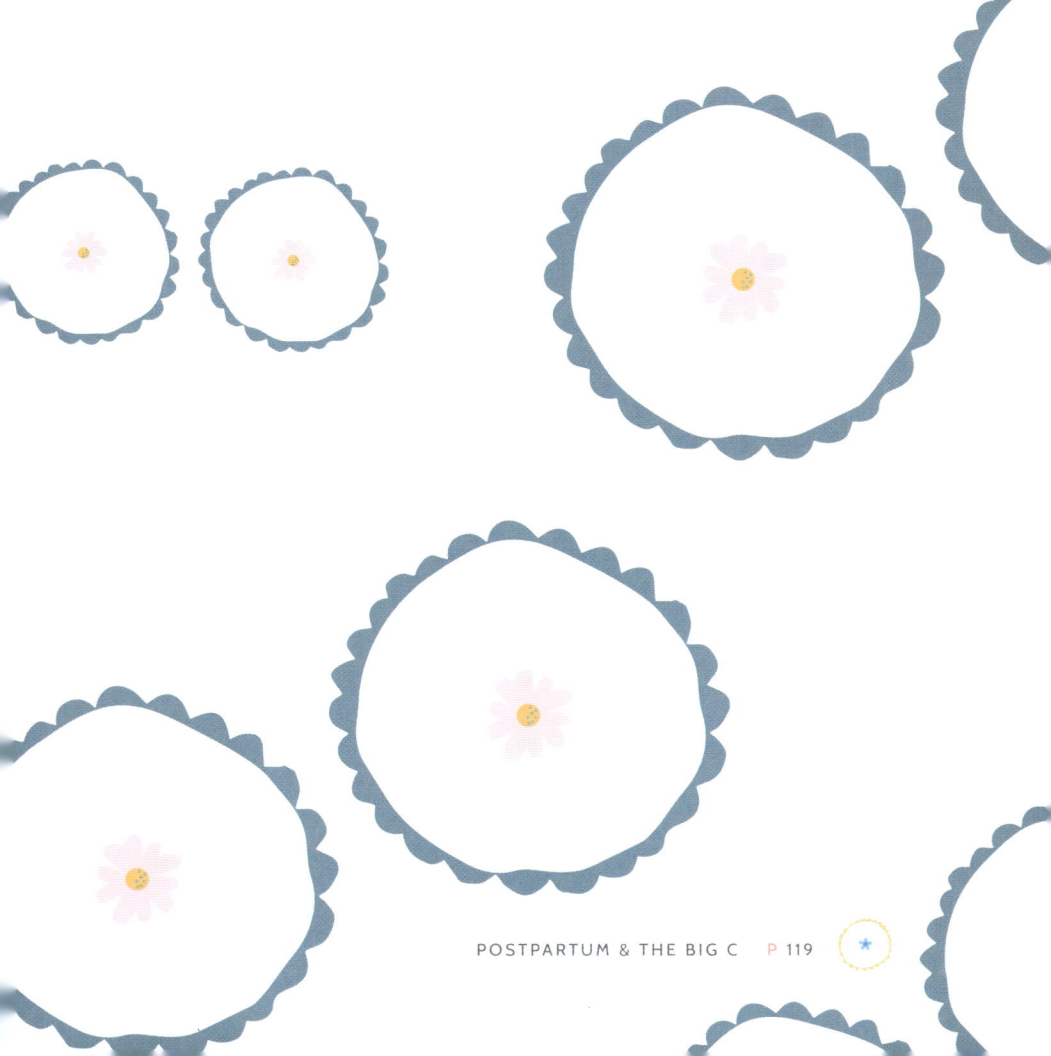

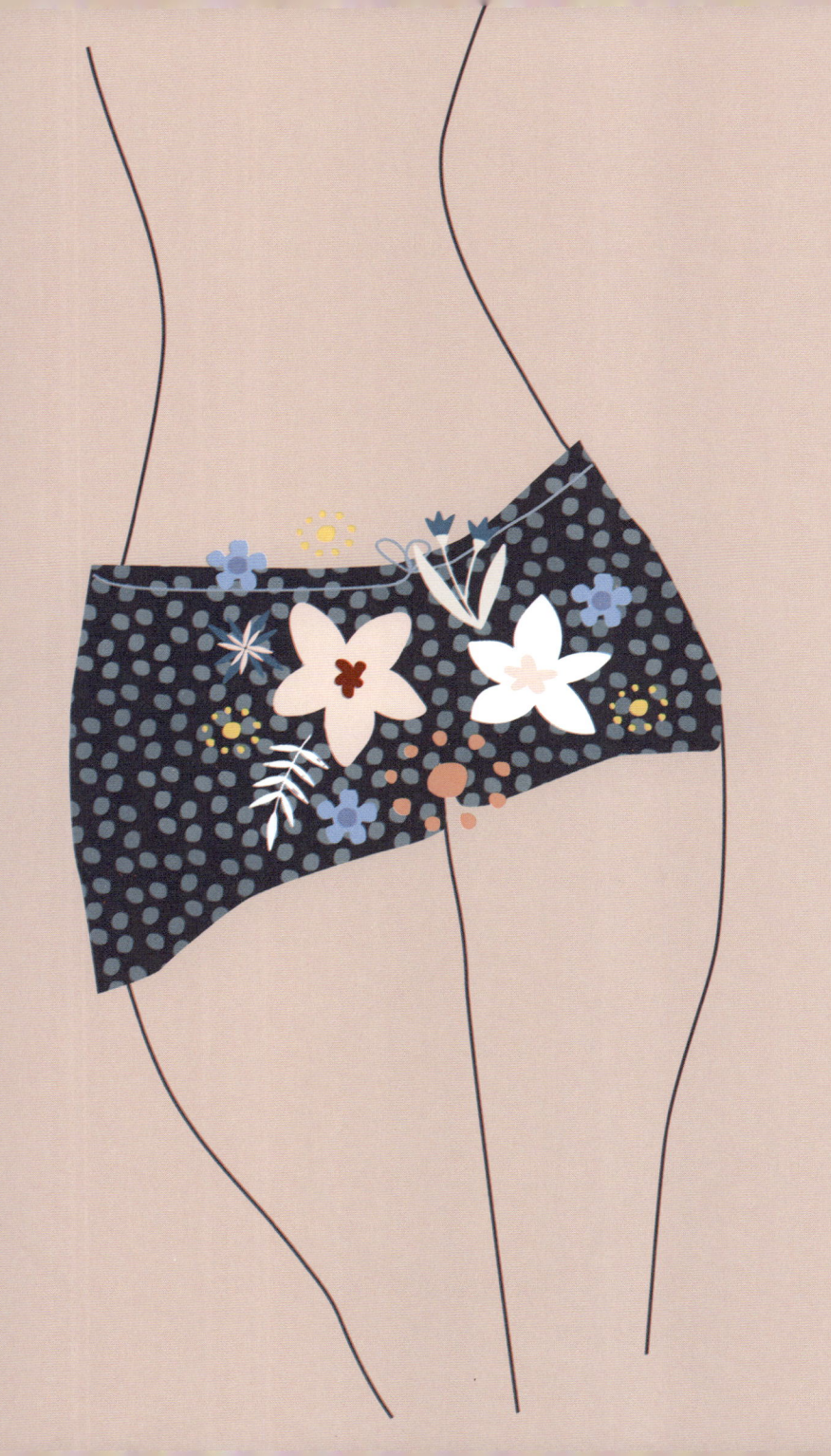

CHAPTER 7
Vanity

Anyone else wondering …

"When can I get a wax again or return to laser? When can I start using that Retinol night cream I paid hundreds for right before I fell pregnant? And when on earth can I ask the pharmacist for something that isn't folic acid, iron or stool softeners?"

After wondering these things does anyone else then think to themselves, "How self-indulgent? I have a new baby to feed & love yet all I can think about is going back to the beautician & taking some Nurofen to numb the pain? Am I that vain?"

Hell no! You are not vain at all. You are well within your rights to feel curious about when you might be ready to regain control over your own body… including the maintenance & pharmaceutical dependence that comes with the territory.

It's not a self-obsessed trait to want to feel good in your own skin. And if people make you feel as if it is, they are not your people. Find new ones.

Out of the curiosities above why don't we start with a very common one; the good old Brazilian Wax or Laser hair removal appointment.

First off, it would be such an unfair judgment to cast on yourself if you deemed any kind of worry about the state of your vagina (or any other part of your body), to be "vain" or "superficial" after having your baby. You are allowed to care & value your appearance when you're a new Mum. For those of you who do, caring about these things doesn't make you silly or petty, or shallow. It makes you human. Not *woman* … human.

With the many movements of late hovering around the subject of female empowerment, there comes an expectation that women should perhaps quit agonising about what they look like and behave in a way that separates them from their sense of femininity. I, for one would like to think that you can do it all.

You can be an empowered, modern day woman and still hope that your vagina, your stomach & your boobs are not completely dictated during pregnancy and labour.

Do I sound nuts? I really hope not as yes I love my brain but I also quite like my body. Shoot me!

So if you are someone who is thinking or perhaps worrying about the day you'll return to your beautician for a waxing or laser appointment, let's dive into this thought because it is of value.

Firstly, if your appointment falls before you return to any kind of intimacy with your partner**, your beautician might be the first person to visit the birthing region after having your baby (other than medical professionals of course) hence any feelings of anxiety. In my eyes, a little anxiety around this appointment is justified. Totally.

All credit to those who don't think twice about it but for others who have thoughts such as the below racing through their heads, why don't we explore the issue from the perspective of a professional beautician?

- ◊ What does it look like now?
- ◊ What if it looks so bad they send me home?
- ◊ Is this going to hurt more than it used to? Or am I now numb from the waist down?
- ◊ Maybe I should just wear trunks from now on? G-strings & Brazilian cuts might be over for me.
- ◊ Did Reece Witherspoon freak out about her waxing appointment after birthing her kids?
- ◊ What about the Queen! Did THE QUEEN share these worries? Wait…. Hang on, were there beauticians back then? Surely waxing The Queen is illegal in London?

◊ F*** F*** F*** F***

◊ Sorry husband, wife, partner, friend. I am now celibate. Bars closed, I'm fencing myself in.

◊ Toodle-oo vagina. Was nice knowing ya!

Let's ease our worries hey? Below we chat to the warm & wonderful beauty therapist & genuine soul queen Tiff (@tiffsmithshiels) from Rona Rituals (@rona_rituals) …

1. If a woman asked you when it was safe to return to waxing (Brazilian/bikini) post-birth (vaginal and or C-Section) what would your advice be?

Firstly I would applaud them for wanting to even make a wax appointment! I then advise & allow them to make an appointment 6 weeks postpartum... just to allow everything to heal best as possible. For the women who have had a C-Section I would definitely avoid waxing until the scar is fully healed & has no sight of scabbing and I'd thoroughly make sure my client is comfortable with me applying pressure & waxing near her scar. And finally I'd ask if she'd had any stitches post-birth & if so - have they dissolved.

It's a very precious area. One that needs to be treated with gentle care.

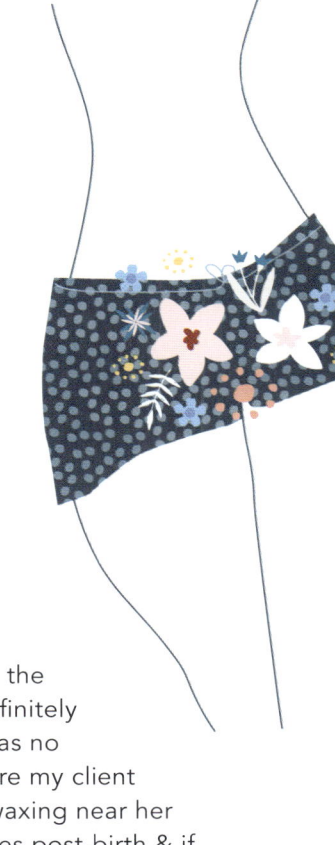

2. If a woman comes to her appointment & she's nervous or shy about what her downstairs region might look like - what do you tell them to calm their nerves?

Again, firstly I'd praise the area as it birthed a human! I mean how phenomenal! Following that would come to validate her feelings (as they're absolutely justified), and remind her that while she may feel a particular way I do not care about what her vulva looks like. I always fully disclose that if at any point she doesn't want to continue the treatment we can absolutely stop at any point. No worry, no judgment.

Personally, I tend to suggest to my clients that if they feel nervous about coming back for a Brazilian (if that is their usual treatment), that it might be a good idea to start with a standard bikini wax. At each appointment moving forward we can work up to a Brazilian.

I care about making sure you are hair free & comfortable.

3. Now tell us the juicy stuff. When it comes to women who have had vaginal births, does their vagina differ vastly?

I honestly have no idea if there is a difference (not that I'm intentionally ever comparing before and after)! Women may feel like there is a variation postpartum but honestly? I can't tell. Some clients have shared with me that their labia has changed & is darker in colour postpartum... but that's it! Nothing scary.

4. Does their downstairs region require a different technique or does it generally take longer to complete?

Post-birth? No! Same vagina. Same hair. BUT I will say that cesarean scarring has to be tendered to with caution and if an episiotomy has been performed it's good for a beautician to be aware of that area as well. So if you just give them the heads up when you make the booking - that is perfect. (It's so funny thinking about all this! These are just the things I just know and have never had to answer or even think about. So clearly ladies - it's all good at our end!! There is absolutely nothing to fear or feel shy about!)

5. For women who are returning to laser hair removal - are there any kind of precautions they should take?

Just be very cautious with any scarring & open wounds. If wounds are still open or very fresh & tender, it's definitely advised to wait to return to waxing or laser until they've fully healed for health & safety reasons.

6. From your experience, are these common worries for women who are returning to the beautician post-birth?

I just feel as though women would feel a little more vulnerable than usual & may also feel nervous about experiencing pain in that area again. I can understand that they could be self-conscious about what their vulva looks like postpartum & perhaps even anxious that I'd judge them. It's absolutely awful to think that women are thinking about themselves in this way!!

In my experience, however, I've found that in general many women are nervous about what their vulva looks like. It's not just the postpartum vulvas ... it's all vulvas! To this day I have NEVER come across a vulva twin. Not one is the same. For all the years I've been waxing I know this but I forget that not all women share in the comfort of this knowledge. Trust me, ladies, they are beautifully unique!

Again, bravo for any babe braving a wax post baby!!

7. When making an appointment for waxing or laser - would you prefer they inform you they've recently had a baby or does it make no difference?

Personally I'd more like to know so that I can offer extra TLC. In terms of scarring once my client is on the table I can make a casual assessment & go over some common postpartum questions with my client. I haven't treated laser for long enough to feel completely comfortable commenting, however I'm sure there would be some standard postpartum protocols - so best to ask your therapist on your phone. Expect no judgment!

8. Is there a reason why women should avoid returning to waxing or laser after their birth? For example, if they're still bleeding, if their stitches have not completely dissolved?

No waxing until 6 weeks postpartum & I wouldn't commit to a booking unless a woman's scarring had fully healed. I don't mind if my client is still bleeding. If she is 100% comfortable that is all that matters to me!

Did you just sigh a sigh of relief? I truly hope so.

Aside from grooming the downstairs region if you want to ask someone to mind the bub while you get your hair done, your brows shaped, your lashes tinted. If you want to get a facial or simply have a longer shower so you can wash your hair & shave your legs ... do it! Your life did not stop the day you welcomed your mini, it simply changed.

Yes, you have to get organised and ask for help. Yes, you might get stuck with guilt pains as let's face it, as much as we shouldn't feel guilty about taking time for ourselves, all Mummas do! If you can do what makes you feel good and find ways to make sure "the old you" doesn't get completely lost in the madness of newborn life you may surprise yourself and uncover a little calmness.

It's perfectly ok to want to look & feel your best. Christ, most of the time it's not even about wanting to look your best, it's just about wanting to look like someone who remembered to shower & brush their teeth. It's not vanity. I repeat it's not vanity. It's simply living.

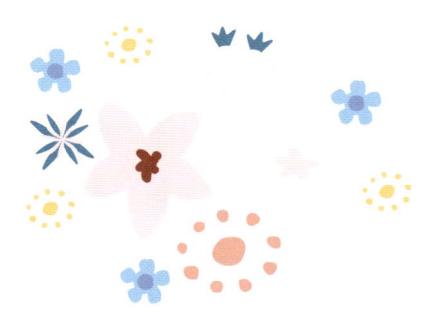

**Please note that when I say "intimacy with your partner" I am very well aware that the term intimacy can mean different things to different people after they give birth. So here I refer to both those who class intimacy as a wild, sweaty romp on the couch … just as much as I refer to those who class intimacy as a fully clothed, friendly foot massage from a safe, non-irritating, and conservative distance.

Letters to myself...

Dear me,

Today I washed my hair & grazed my knee. I must remember to move that basket I keep tripping on in the dark. I managed to rock the baby into the deepest sleep just after my breakfast. It was the perfect way to finish my coffee & start their day, in restful silence. And then just 13 short minutes later, I heard the baby wake. It wasn't enough sleep. I told the baby that. They didn't care, I didn't argue. So now with my clean hair that is still damp and heavy, and my stinging knee, I sit and patiently yet impatiently wait for the minutes to pass. How many minutes you may ask? Lots. I need a whole collection of minutes that feel longer than the last to pass before I'll have the energy to stand up once again and rock the baby back to sleep. While I sit here, if you could quieten your chatter, that would be kind. I know you've been reading the sleep books and I understand that this hiccup doesn't fit in. Sometimes things don't fit in. Things stray, towards the good and the tough. So let's just wait until we stray towards a kinder direction. It'll be so wonderful when we arrive there. Let's use this time to dream of it. x

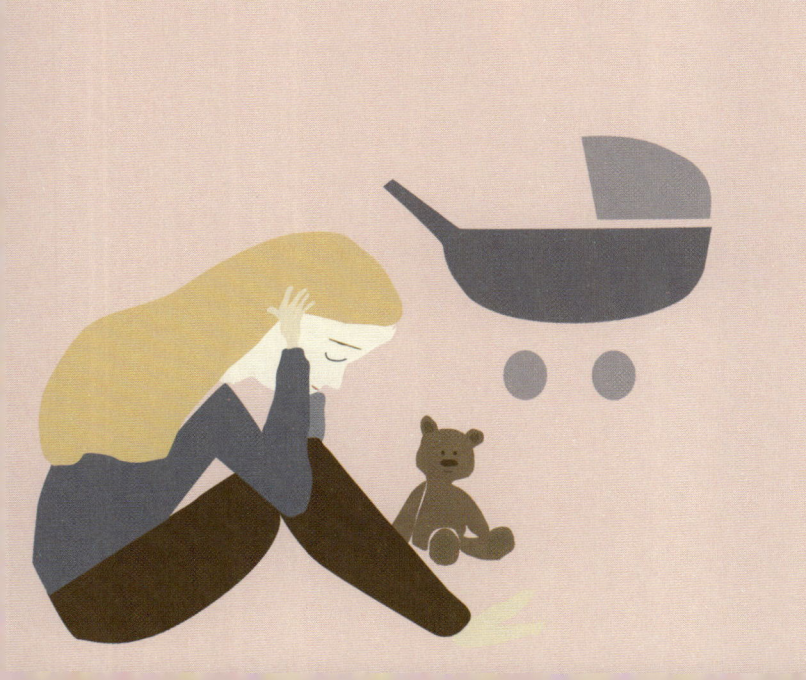

CHAPTER 8

Mr. Guilt

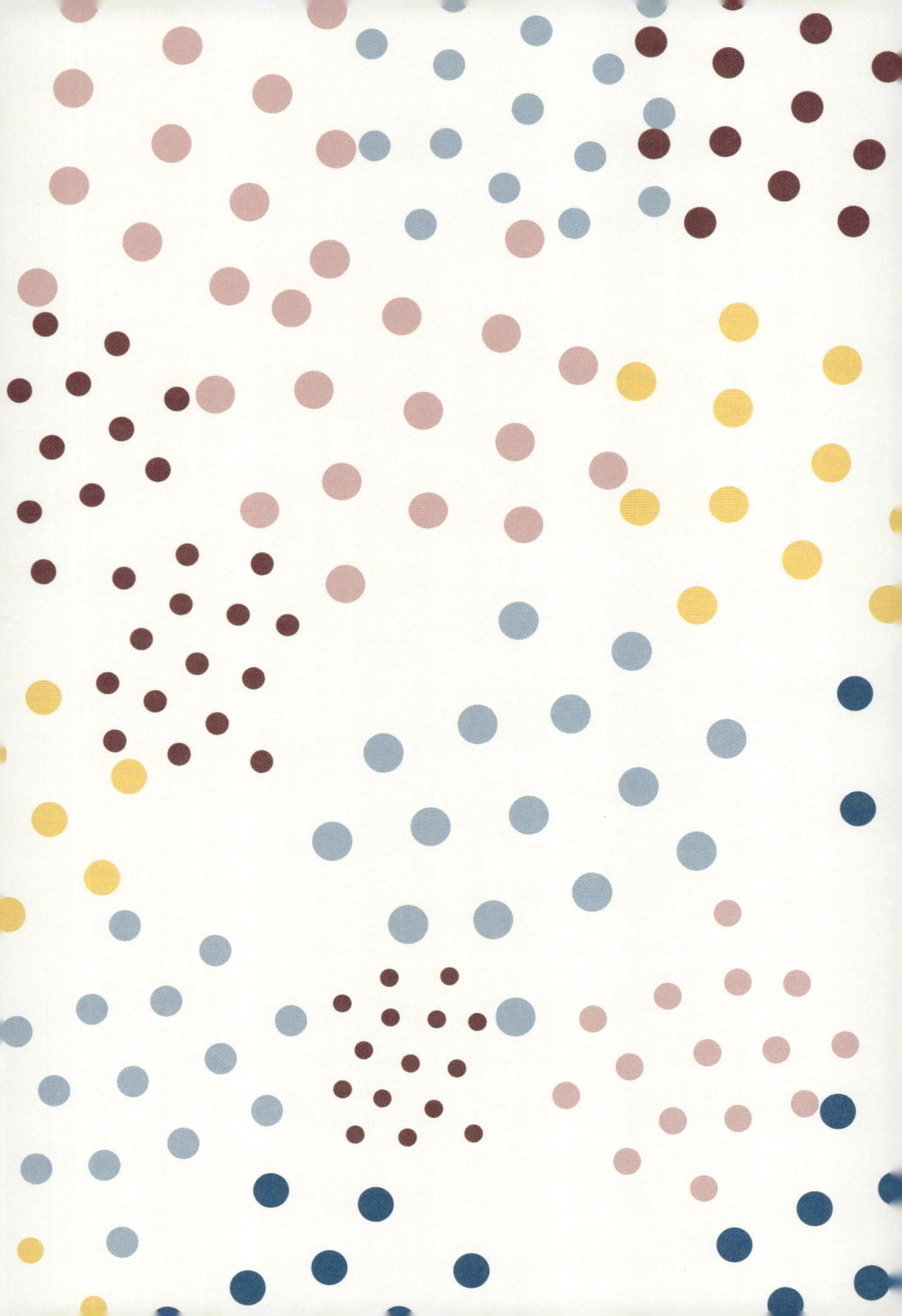

Mr. Guilt ... the grouch, the grinch. What a dickhead.

Mothers feel guilty for SO many things following the birth of a child. Maybe not all of us but many of us. Even though we love our children more than life itself, don't think it's uncommon to have moments where you feel overwhelmed and genuinely frustrated by the countless ways a baby changes your life.

Remember all of that time you don't have anymore? The freedom you surrendered the day you left the hospital? Remember when you had control over your own body? What about that time when you knew how to not put the right shoe on the left foot four times in a row, or the days when you wore clothes that weren't stained by milk. Remember your friends?

Who remembers a time when 4 hours of consecutive sleep didn't deserve a bottle of French champagne, a group text to the entirety of your family, and an almighty scream from the rooftop, "MY BABY IS A GENIUS! HE'S NOT BROKEN AFTER ALL!"

... and the days when you could operate a vehicle alone? As in drive to the shops to buy eggs and glad wrap without having to recite the frantic words, "NEARLY THERE DARLING. NEARLY THERE. NEARLY THERE!!" Mate. Those days feel like they were part of another lifetime. And didn't we live on the edge back then? I mean, driving a car alone? All by ourselves? If that's not luxury, I don't know what is.

Remember the life and times before you were known as Mumma?

Before parenting became a new role in your life of course, you knew to expect changes. But the level of change is incomprehensible. The actuality of the changes to your day-to-day existence is spectacularly far off what you assumed. Right? Nothing can truly prepare you for the arrival of your new housemate. A socially awkward person who likes to glue themselves to your body at the most inconvenient of hours. Newborns have some serious issues with being alone.

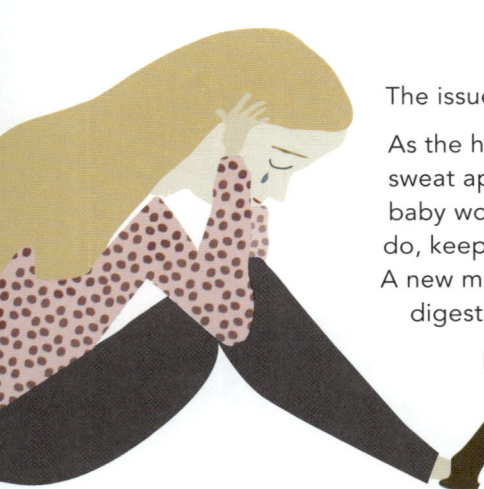

The issue being, they are repulsed by it.

As the hours tick over and little beads of sweat appear on your forehead because your baby won't do what the book said it would do, keep calm. It's ok. The moment will pass. A new moment will come. An easier, more digestible moment will find you.

For now, just do your very best to cope. Try to focus on putting one foot in front of the other. If you can do that you're doing incredibly well. Transitioning to motherhood is ... it's beyond the depth of language.

If and when you crave your old life, Fair Enough. If you want to sue the author of the sleep guide that makes you sweat with a complex blend of genuine panic & infuriation when it's mentioned on the mothers group WhatsApp, then I advise you Google a lawyer and trust their fees will steer you out of a court proceeding.

If you feel ashamed & as if you're unraveling with guilt because you don't enjoy every single moment. You feel like all the other Mums so affectionately talk about the "newborn bubble of love"... yet your bubble popped last week & left a giant bitch of a puddle on the floor for you to mop up. It's not just you having these surges of culpability. There is a plethora of other Mums feeling the same way. I wish we all remembered this as much as we remember that once again, we forgot to buy Napisan at the supermarket. Mothers guilt is a savage emotion.

The second you surrender to guilt or let it consume your mind and thoughts tell yourself to get rational and to get rational quickly. It'll defeat you otherwise. Just for now, imagine that guilt is an irritating, nosy neighbour. Let's call him Mr. Guilt from down the road.

Mr. Guilt keeps popping around to your house to complain that your car is parked too far off the curb, your lemon tree is hanging over their fence, your lawns need to be mowed, your dog keeps weeing on their lawn, your TV is far too loud around 6pm. Mr. Guilt is the type of neighbour who is always going to have a problem with you because he has nothing else to do. And worse yet, Mr. Guilt is the type of neighbour who ain't going anywhere.

Stop answering your door. We are all proud people & of course we all want our lawns to look lovely every single day of the week .. but let's get real. Sometimes our lawns become jungles. Just like sometimes our lives become circuses. And you know what? Who f***ing cares.

Mr. Guilt is dickhead. You are a new Mum doing your best to get through the day. You win.

So when these icky thoughts enter your mind, do something to distract yourself. If you're lying in bed listen to a fun Podcast. If you're rocking your baby to sleep start singing a song. If you are at the hairdressers - get that small talk going! Get busy, get loud and smother any sounds of cynicism.

But please remember if you do feel guilty and have days where you are too tired to get loud and busy it's normal. We all get slapped with some kind of guilt from time to time. It's not a sign of weakness or a sign you're being an overbearing worrywart. It's just another human emotion we are all faced with.

Skim through the below if you feel like you need something to relate to. Sometimes simply relating to others can lift a huge weight from your shoulders.

If I've written it, I've felt it. Trust me.

- ◊ Your friends & their babies are so great at arranging play dates in the park but with your work schedule or just your flat mood today, you feel like you're always unable to make it. You stay home worrying about depriving your baby of social experiences while also being a shitty friend.
= Guilt.

- ◊ A load of clean washing has sat in the washing basket since the Tuesday before last. You're more tempted to chuck it all out and just buy new clothes. Then you think of landfill, then you think of people with so little & then you remember you're an adult.
= Guilt.

- ◊ You've cooked dinner for the last 3 nights and you feel as though you deserve a medal, a night off in a 5-star hotel and 2 hour massage followed by a facial. Then you remember the dinners you cooked... Tuna salad, tuna salad, and the night before that it was Gin and oats.
= Guilt.

- ◊ You know your partner wants to have sex but you're too tired because you've lugged a small Michelin man on your hip all day.
= Guilt.

- ◊ You go off to an exercise class in the morning & take the longest route home because you just crave a bit of time to yourself. You know your partner has to get to work & your baby needs a feed but you just want another kilometer of silence.
= Guilt.

- You go to the "boutique grocery" almost every day to buy the 7 out of 10 things you forgot to buy at the supermarket. It costs 20 times the price & your items always seem to be a quarter of the size but you do it anyway.
  = Guilt.

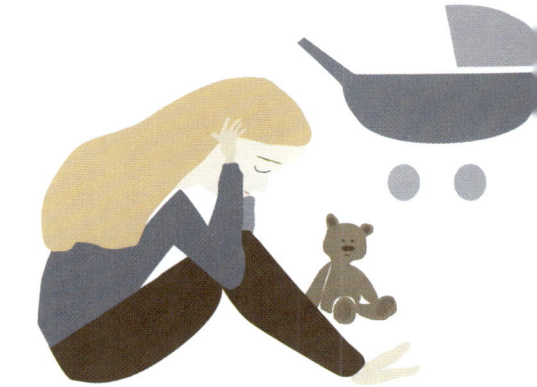

- While you're at the "boutique grocery," you buy your partner a surprise treat to brighten their day. You eat the surprise treat on the way home & hide the wrapper, not to hide the evidence but to hide your shame.
  = Guilt.

- You let your baby cry on their play mat for longer than usual. Not because you don't care about their current conniption and their stress over the fact they can't find Spot, but because today your ears have taken a Mental Health Day. You hear nothing but the white noise that now haunts you.
  = Guilt.

- You shut your eyes and sleep when the baby sleeps leaving 5 text messages yet to be read and replied to.
  = Guilt.

- You try so hard to keep your little one away from digital objects for as long as possible but today you give in. "Have my phone, here's the remote control, have Dad's laptop. Whatever you want, take it. TAKE IT ALL!"
  = Guilt.

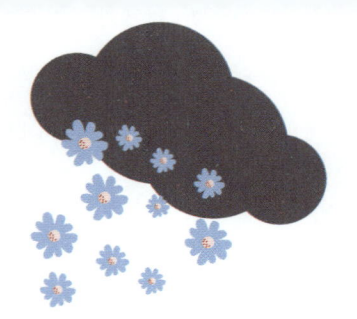

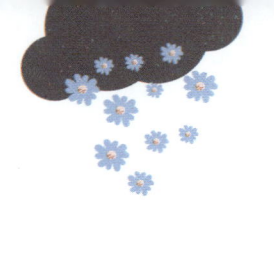

◊ The Instagram babies are dressed in white linen and various shades of olive and terracotta. They eat organic sardines with avocado while sitting on a peaceful white beach. Your naked baby is on the floor, eating a paper plate & sucking on a peg.
= Guilt.

◊ It's 11am on a Wednesday. You see so many people rushing from meeting to meeting as they make the economy go round & round. You're out for your 3rd walk for the day listening to a Podcast about The Bachelorette.
= Guilt.

◊ It's 5.03pm and you've already finished your 5 o'clock glass of wine.
= Guilt.

◊ You pat your baby's little back & stroke their warm forehead when they're teething, tired, and in need of their Mumma. You yawn uncontrollably & wish for someone to rub your back.
= Guilt.

◊ You coat your baby's delicate skin in lovely oils to make them feel relaxed. You feel calm, in love & so at peace. Then you remember your girlfriend who is struggling with their baby's reflux issues and hasn't slept in 3 days.
= Guilt.

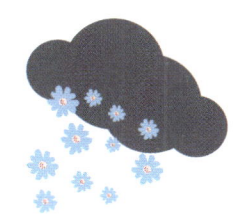

You adore your baby.

You love them unconditionally.

You miss them when they sleep.

You worry your heart will implode when you hear them giggle.

You promise to do whatever it takes to ensure their health, happiness & comfort is never compromised … and yep.

Guilt still manages to rear its ugly head because even though you promise to do all the right things by them, you know you haven't done them yet. You might stuff up … you might get it wrong.

Do you see?

Even when you're doing your very best mum-ing. Even when you are exceeding your own expectations. Even when you finally admit to yourself that being a Mum is a hard role to take on but you're coping really well … you feel guilty.

And the big fat cherry on top?

During all of this you always seem to feel guilty that there is another woman out there, another amazing woman, who may never have the chance to experience what you're experiencing because for one reason or another she is unable to have her own baby. You are one of the lucky ones while they are dealt an unfair joker.

Guilt will always find you and it can smother you.

For many mothers guilt is not so much about their baby but more about their other relationships. For the mothers who choose to take maternity leave & therefore can't contribute as much to the mortgage there's a sense of letting your partner down.

Some Mums may question themselves & their abilities when comparing their choice to work or not to work based on what their sister, friend, colleague or their own Mum chose to do during pregnancy & postpartum. Then there are the Mums who decide to return to work earlier than anticipated because they miss their sense of purpose in the workplace. Even though it's a choice they make, they feel as though their femininity or their maternal instincts are reoriented towards that of a less caring mother.

On the topic of choices & as touched on above some women are robbed of the choice to fall pregnant naturally and go on to endure months to years of fertility treatments. They invest every ounce of hope and emotion into conceiving a child & exhaust their body while doing whatever it takes to become a mother.

Then the magical day comes! They fall pregnant & 9 months later they hold their cherished bundle in their arms … yet they're crying? Just like all new mothers, they are tired, uncomfortable, confused, and wishing they could escape back to their pre-baby lives for just one day to rest and recoup. But how dare they be anything but grateful? They longed for this for so long and now it's here and what … it's too much? You have to be kidding!

If this is you, dry your tears. You are not ungrateful. You are a wonderful person who moved oceans to bring life into the world. You are the strongest of all.

And finally, the last of the list that doesn't even scratch the surface of reasons behind a mother's guilt … when you have coffee with a friend & reminisce about the morning you had. Balancing a deadline, dealing with a nappy explosion, all the while having had no sleep the night before. The friend so kindly says, "I don't know how you do it? You're amazing."

You sit opposite & think, "Now I'm the dickhead. She must think I'm fishing for a compliment because I did 2 measly things at once! She has 3 kids under six & she brought home-made hummus to the last playgroup with a home-grown lemon to squeeze on top, and her shirt appears to be IRONED!"

Where is guilt NOT!?! Where? As I said, it will always find you.

At times it feels impossible to ease up on the self-deprecation. Distracting yourself & moving on from the feeling is one way to power through. Just keep moving forward & shh'ing out the unwanted thoughts. Or perhaps another way around the guilt, or just a way to take the edge off, is to look at things from another person's perspective?

If someone says YES to catching up at a cafe near your place yet far from theirs …

If someone OFFERS to drop you off a coffee …

If you enrol your bub in daycare because you CHOOSE to do so …

If you have a glass of wine WHILE catching up on emails …
… allow your guilt to exist as gratitude.

Even if you sit on your phone while hiding in the loo & live vicariously through someone else's life for 10 minutes … it is OK! Whatever gets you through a moment of hardship.

If you have your first shower at 3pm, if you eat your babies snacks, if you forget to buy toilet paper at the shops and use a box of tissues for the week … it is OK.

You are OK. Your baby is OK.

OK?

Shut the door on Mr. Guilt & hang a sign on your gate that simply says, PISS OFF, I'M BUSY.

P 144   AFTERWARDS

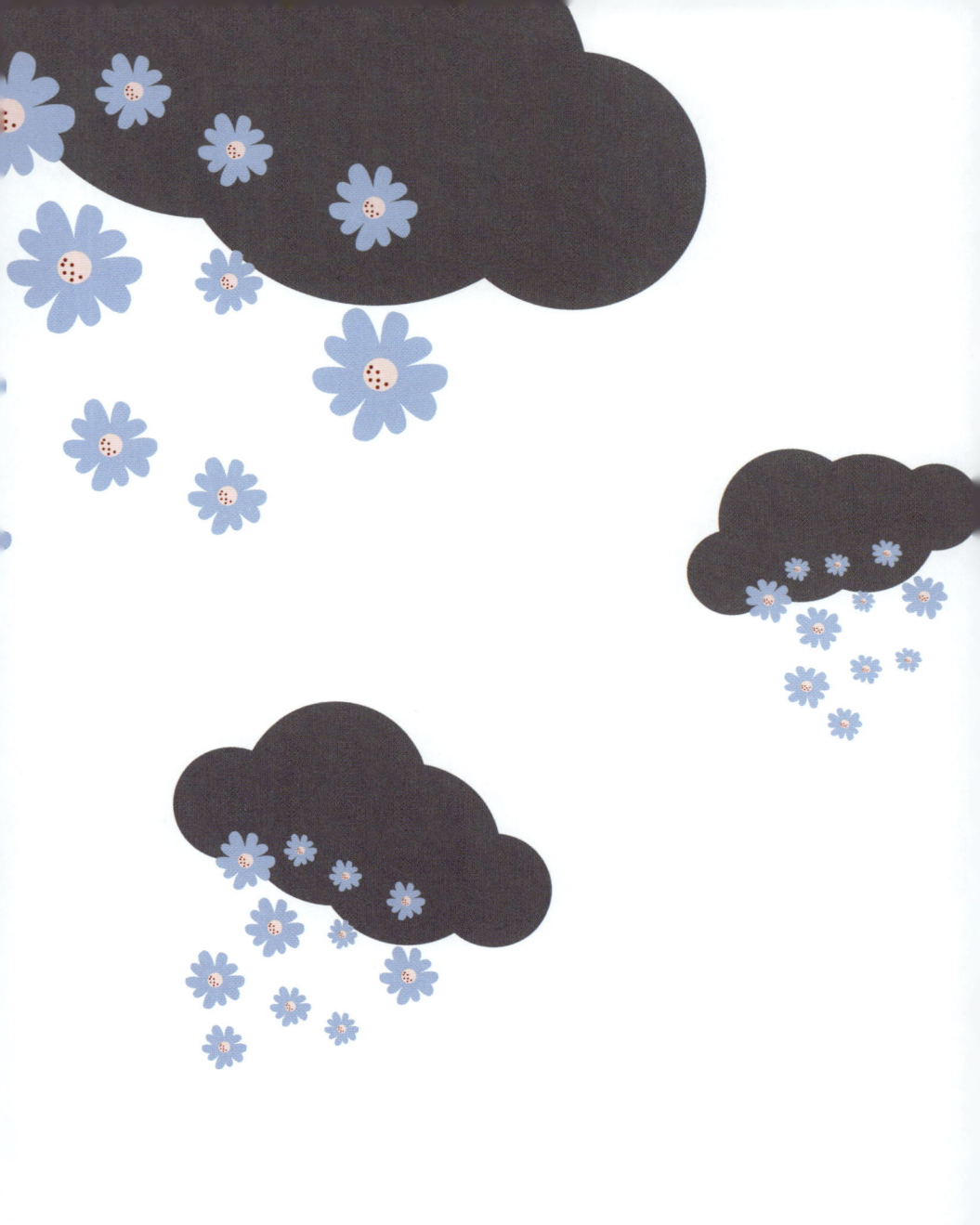

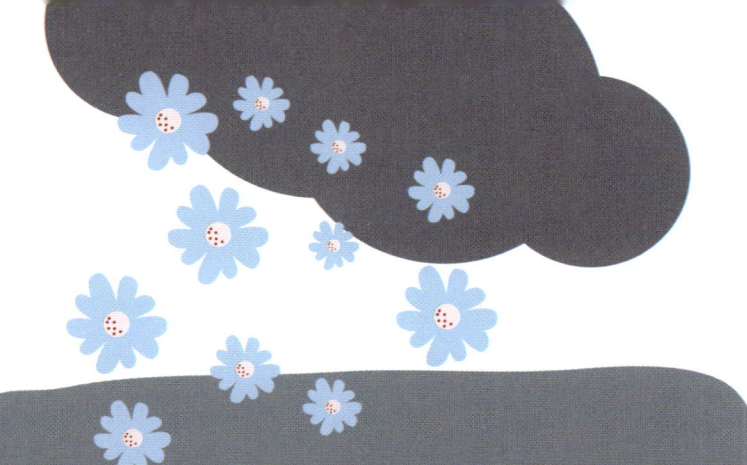

To finish up on guilt, let's take a moment to explore the term milestone, as this word seems to very easily send new Mums into a cyclone of worry. And worry can quickly erupt into guilt. Our midwife Sophie Outhwaite explains the term below for those who are unsure.

The term Milestones gets Mums wound up & perhaps even a little too obsessive with what their babies should be doing & when. Can you offer some practical & rational advice around this?

Milestones are based on the average age children learn new skills and behaviours, so they are useful for recognising the signs of atypical development and seeking early intervention if it is necessary, but that's about it. Australian babies have a busy schedule of vaccinations and checks in their first few years of life, so if you're worried about your baby's development for any reason use these appointments to talk to your GP or Child Health Nurse.

quick hack

BE READY, BE SAFE, BE RESPONSIBLE

Nearly every household with a new baby will have an experience or an isolated incident that will create intense panic & unforgettable fear. An incident where for one reason or another, you'll fear for your bubs safety & their health. Infants are so incredibly precious & vulnerable, and as a first time parent you'll be hyper-vigilant when it comes to their protection.

When & if something goes wrong, and god forbid it ever does, do yourself and your family the greatest favour on earth and be ready. Have a look at some tips below and then jump onto this great website for anything you may need; The Safety Store Australia (www.safetystoreaustralia.com.au)

◊ Organise a Baby First Aid Course. Most hospitals in each state will offer a 1 or 2 day intensive course. Alternatively, you can book a private course where a certified professional in the field travels to your place of residence & goes through critical subjects such as CPR/resuscitation, choking, burns, bleeding, poison, bites & stings and how to operate an automatic defibrillator. The latter is a great idea, as automatic defibrillators are now commonly found in gyms, pools, shopping centres, offices & other public areas.

I cannot recommend or encourage this tip highly enough. I participated in a one day course with about

7 other couples, all who had newborns and/or toddlers. It was intense, eye opening & worth every second and cent. *Professionals recommend you re-do a course of this nature every year or two.

◊ Ensure you have a well stocked & up to date First Aid Kit (or a few scattered across the home & cars). Your First Aid Kit should come with saline water, burns assistance (Google & purchase Burnshield dressings), plasters, gauze and dressings (in a whole range of shapes & sizes), instant icepacks, antibacterial swabs and spray, shock blankets, eye pads, gloves, scissors, splinter probes, a triangle bandage (i.e. a sling). The list could go on … & the price will range between $70-$150 per kit. This is a game changing investment.

◊ Get Filing. Create a file full of your emergency contacts, your bubs medical history and any other paperwork that needs to be kept safely & on hand. The birth certificate, important test results or information regarding any allergies & other conditions. Mum & Dad's Medicare numbers (including the expiry dates), drivers license details, passport details and anything else that may be required as proof of identity.

If you ever need to jet off to the hospital in a moment of swift panic, grab the file knowing it contains everything you might need and go. Alternatively, if someone is watching your baby and calls you in a panic, instruct them to grab the file and go.

◊ Dedicate a place in your home to visually display emergency contact numbers. Mum, Dad, Grandparents, emergency services, the poison hotline, the GP, a friend or neighbour. Maybe even throw 000 on the list for anyone who may be inclined to dial the ol' 911. Panic = irrational thinking = silly mistakes.

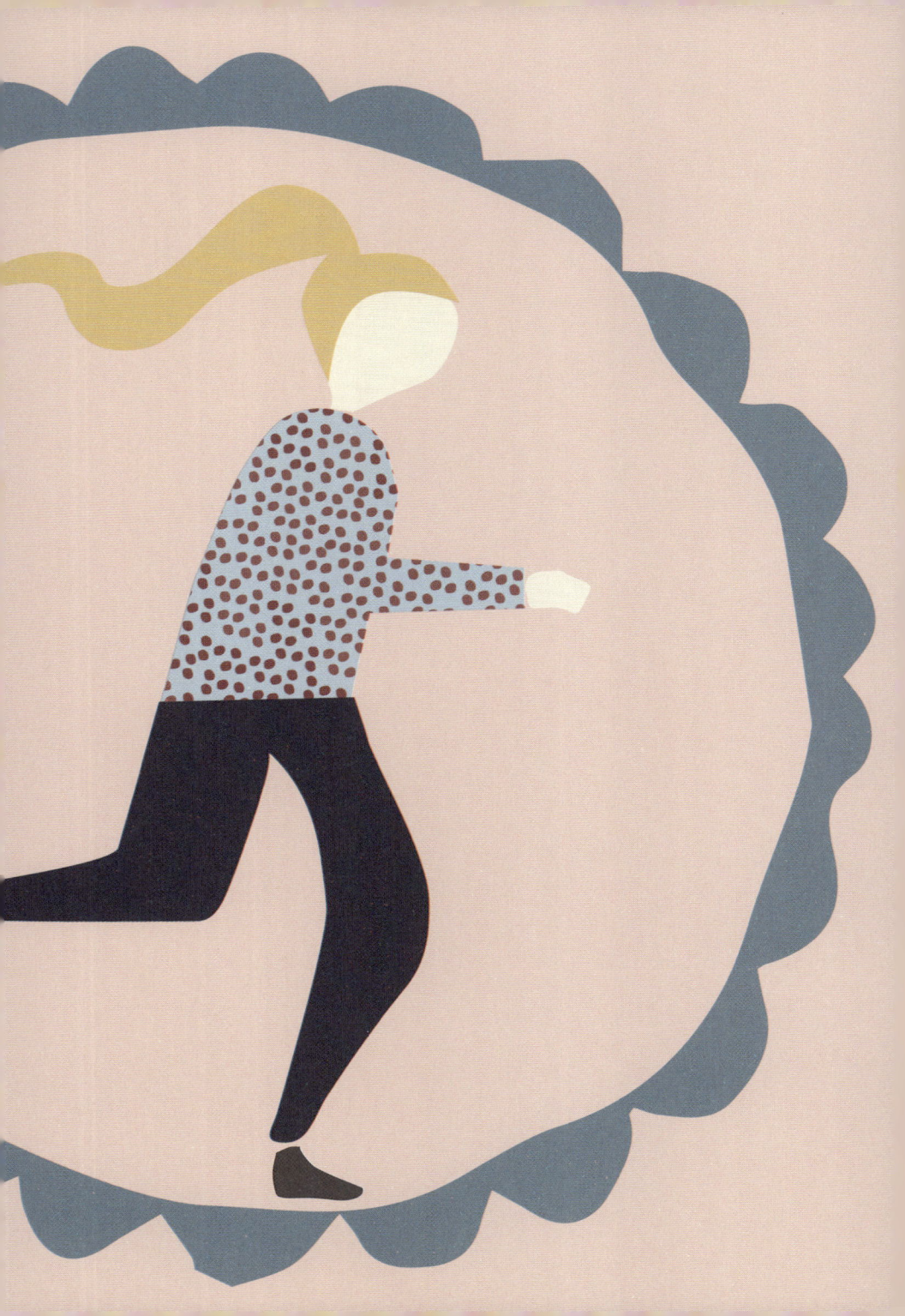

CHAPTER 9

boredom

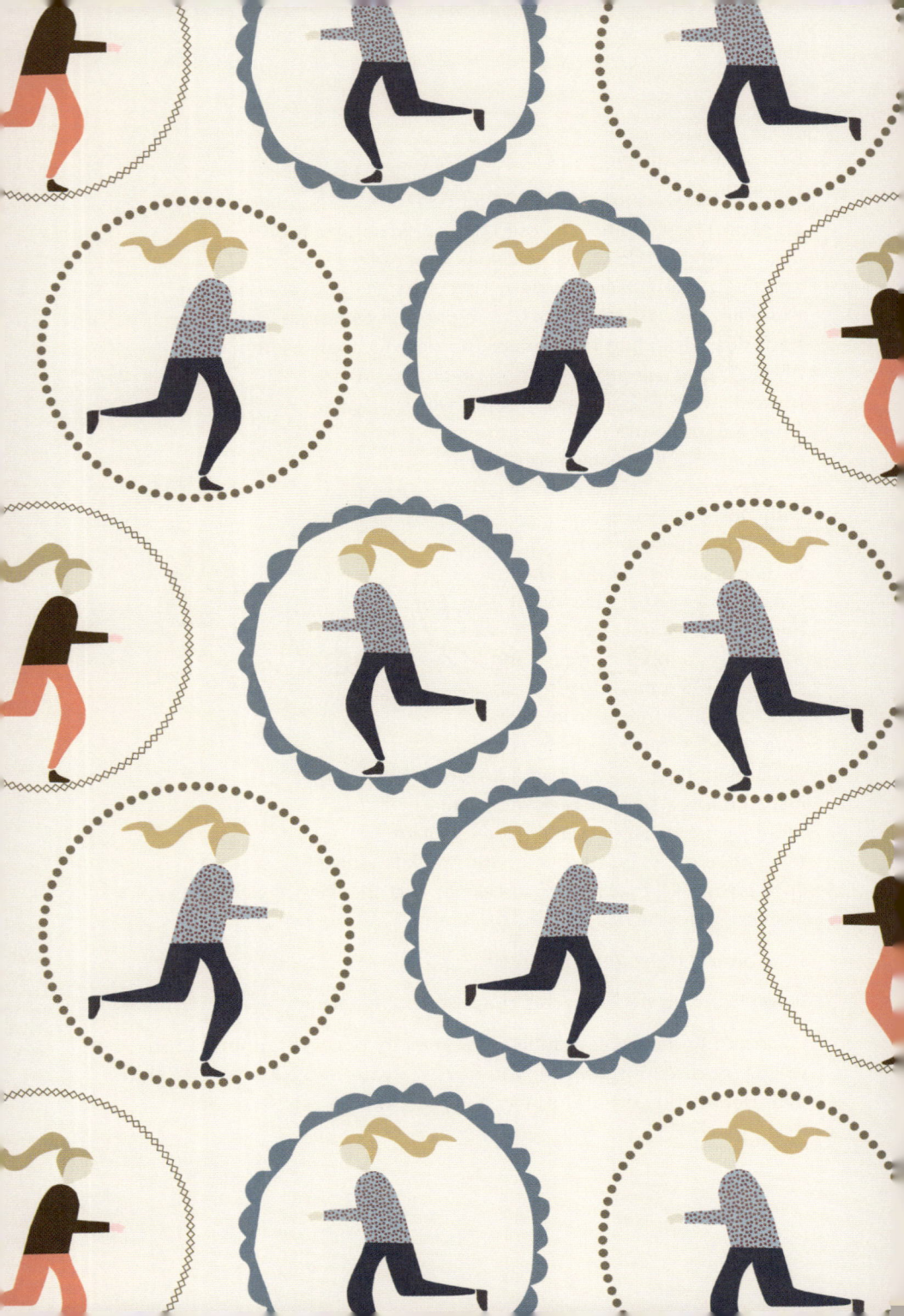

Doing the following …

Folding the washing, soaking stained clothes, changing nappies, emptying bins, pumping your boobs, blitzing up food, picking up toys, wiping down bench tops & sticky fingers, packing the baby bag, unpacking the baby bag, sterilising bottles, getting the pram in & out of the car, changing the white noise machine batteries, repeating the phrase "no darling, thats Mummy's phone", practising gratitude when coating a rosy buttocks with Bepanthem, weeing with a small audience, transforming the task of unpacking the dishwasher into a pantomime performance, exploring with Dora, guessing how much the big rabbit loves the small rabbit & finding Spot fifty times a day (even the newborns know that Spot is in the basket!), loosing your keys only to find them in your other hand, mopping up milk drops, reheating your coffee 19 times, convincing your partner that crying doesn't always signify a leap … sometimes it just signifies a baby is present, wasting money on concealers because they claim to remove dark circles, destroying the kitchen to find a Tupperware lid that fits the container and checking the clock to ask yourself, "How is it ONLY 10.37am?" …

… is boring right. Am I wrong?

If you don't agree - skip this chapter. You're a saint.

Failing to find complete fulfillment in every ounce of motherhood will never discount the love you have for your baby. Nor will it ever deem you ungrateful. You might be willing & able to do "it all" but that doesn't mean you have to wipe up baby vomit while thinking to yourself, "I am so blessed to be here." You can wipe up that baby vomit thinking, "this is disgusting. I would like to be anywhere but here right now," and still be an incredible mother. Of course you can!

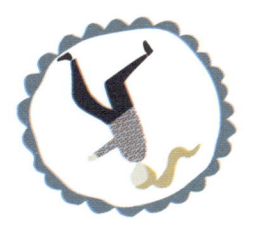

There are parts of motherhood that are mundane, monotonous and boring. Just like in any other job there are going to be elements you'd prefer to ignore. Admitting that the highlight of your day was brushing your teeth is to be expected when your baby is in a blob stage (a beautiful blob stage of course).

Unfortunately we don't all have the Mary Poppins carpet bag of tricks. Most of us just have a combination of a nappy bag and unpacked grocery bags. On top of this however we all have friends and gadgets and minds and imaginations!

On the days you feel bored & underutilized do whatever you can to find the joy in the downtime as it needs to be said … there are going to be many more slow, mundane and dare I say boring days ahead. Many more. Navigating your way through these days is what you need to focus on right now.

Listen to a Podcast and learn something new. Watch trashy TV for the first time in your life to see what all the fuss is about. Find a few wine bottles and do some arm weights, walk the neighbourhood & find your dream home. Clean out your wardrobe, write that business plan you've always wanted to write. Indulge in the days when you have nothing else to do but feed your baby, hold your baby, love your baby.

If your baby is a little older & has graduated from blob to rolling blob to crawling mini-human to walking/borderline toddler … your days won't be so easy to indulge in the downtime. The downtime? What downtime? You'll be busy. But even with busyness comes boringness!

It's fine to admit that.

…

Some women absolutely cherish the role of being a Mumma at home. They thrive in an environment where they so effortlessly transform the space into a place of nurture & solace. When their house is quiet and no one is around except for themselves and their little one, they're perfectly content. They have patiently pined for this.

Regardless of the state of the house, the size of the washing pile & the height of the dishes, they are unfazed. Whether everything is schmick or in complete disarray they glide through the day & the night with a natural sense of control and ease.

Household chores are not always a bag of fun for everyone, gosh no. However there are people out there (myself included), who lean a little to the OCD side. Everything has a place. These Mummas like their environment to be neat & orderly so that every morning they wake up to a space they can make sense of.

Every night they fluff pillows, put everything away, wipe the bench tops & declutter the desk. Despite the day they've had with the baby, with work & with life in general, they prefer things to be tidy. It keeps them sane & energised.

When the baby is awake the house is welcome to exhibit itself as if it's a rampageous circus. But when the baby naps Mumma gets her space back. Some Mums may like to nap when their baby naps others may like to tidy. Whatever the choice, whatever works, whatever allows Mum to cope.

These types of Mums will surely have a thick skin by now anyway. For the entirety of their pregnancy other mothers would have told them as often as possible, "Just you wait, you have no idea what's ahead of you!"… "You see everything in this room? It ALL must go!" … "Your aversion to things that are not well spaced will be your demise." … aka You Are Deluded.

Take the comments of this nature with a grain of salt as it's all hearsay, highly subjective and total bullocks to be honest.

Every mothers journey is different. Every baby is different. Whatever the choice, whatever works, whatever allows Mum to cope.

Let her do her … **however meticulous she may be.**

BOREDOM   P 155

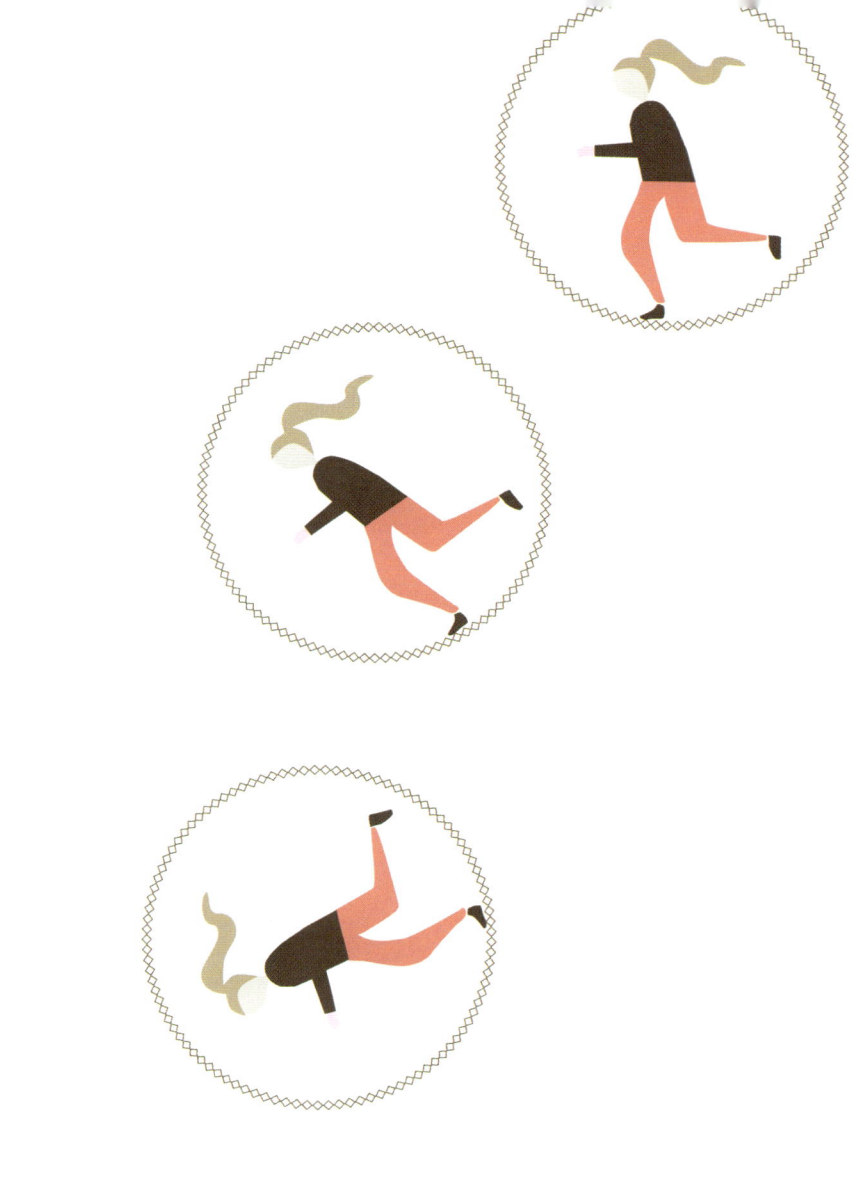

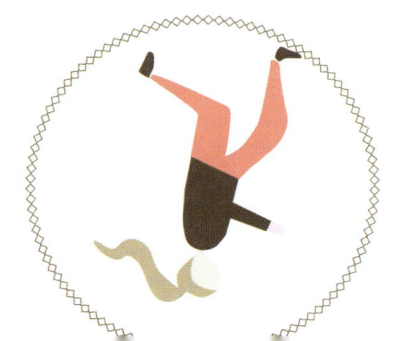

Letters to myself...

Dear me,

How good is life? And hot, soapy showers... how good are hot, soapy showers? x

PS. Today I discovered that there is a line in Magic Beach that doesn't rhyme. I've read it over and over... while this annoys me, it will always remain my very favourite book.

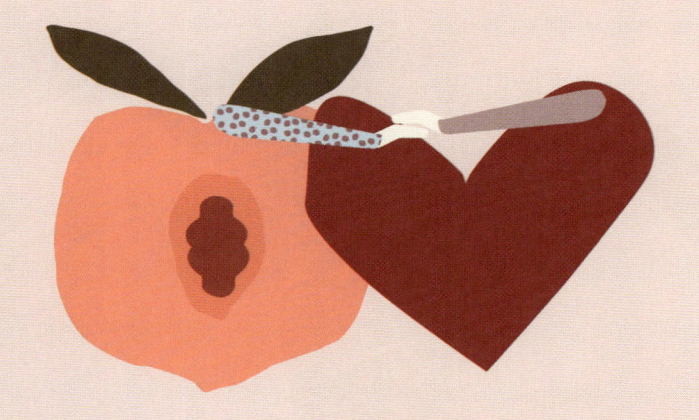

CHAPTER 10

Healing

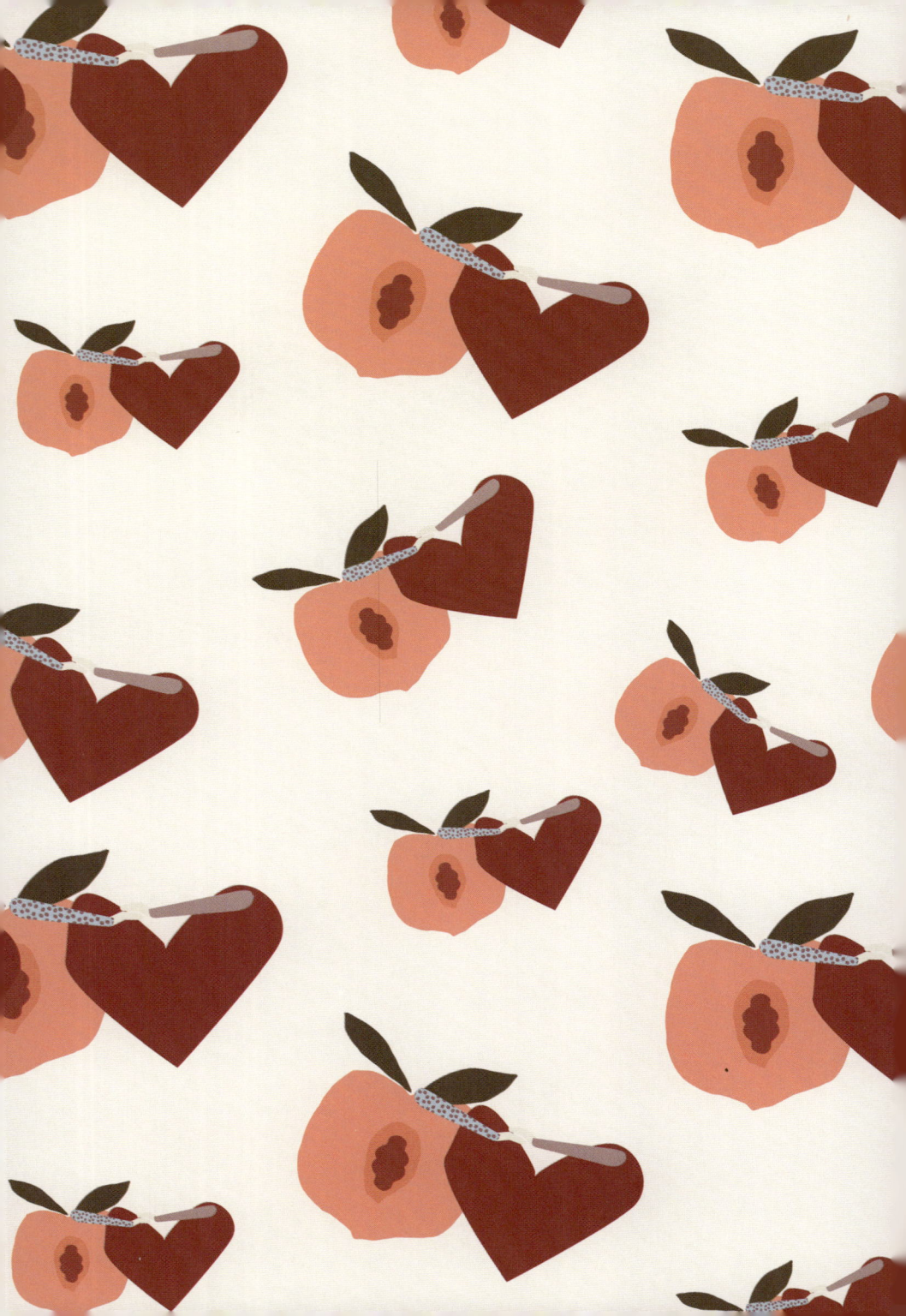

The transition from *me* to *mother* is beyond language. The world shifts, what you used to see clearly has now blurred and your potential to feel compassion, protectiveness, patience, and empathy has expanded from your heart, into your lungs, your skin, your mind, the entirety of your being. You are all consumed. Your normal is new & unrecognisable yet oddly familiar. Your time is shared, your hands are forever busy. It's a massive adjustment & one that may benefit from prioritising the healing process.

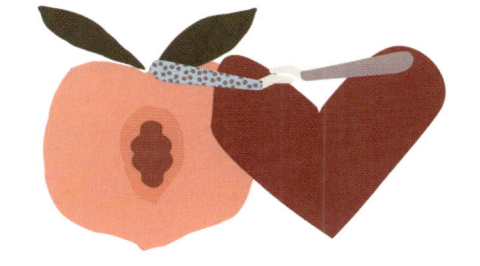

The postnatal journey is a one-way ticket. You never return to the life you lived before you became Mumma. You move forward & go beyond where you thought possible. Without significant warning you veer into a side street that you'll follow along from now on having no real clue where it's going to take you. How exciting is that!?! How magical! Well maybe to some …

Personally, much of the above is horrifically terrifying. I'm a routine kinda gal. I like to know what's happening from the moment I open my eyes in the morning to when I flop back into bed. I like a plan, a schedule, a goal to aim for. I am not spontaneous and surprises are not something I naturally warm towards. Good gosh, don't I sound like a bag of laughs!! I am the LIFE of the party … the well organised, not overly loud party … planned by a party planner who comes with an oversupply of napkins and leaves room in the budget for post party cleaning.

But with routine comes control and with control comes mental ease and a state of calm. I don't doubt for a second that some women reading this will understand what I mean. Some of us are somewhat frightened by the unknown because it removes the ability to prepare.

For many new Mums this fear can stretch far beyond what they're able to cope with. Life can sink into a very dark place at an alarmingly quick rate. While you think you can just label it as a dose of "The Baby Blues" if the blues don't pass and you feel the sting worsening, it's time for you to seek help. In Australia, more than 1 in 7 Mums & up to 1 in 10 Dads* will feel this way ... and the feeling is not isolated to just the newborn phase, nor does it only present itself after the first baby. Postnatal depression is an insidious beast which can occur at any point and it really does warrant professional help. Just like an unwelcome cockroach, postnatal depression isn't phased how it finds it's host. It is not discriminatory nor does it worry about the fear, the shame or the disgust it projects onto those who are forced to look it in the eye. You don't have to bear the presence of the roach, nor do you have to bear the presence of postnatal depression. Find the support available & swat it the hell away.

POSTNATAL DEPRESSION & POSTNATAL ANXIETY

When you become a Mumma for the first time parts of you (of everyone!) will break every once in a while. Let's be honest here shall we? Yes, we can all be brave, strong, and resilient but it's also nice, to be honest, & shine light on those days where we can't help but feel like a bag of wet cement. Heavy & stuck. Some Mummas however will be haunted by this feeling for weeks or months on end. It'll start to blind them.

If anyone was desperately waiting for a chapter on Postnatal Depression (PND) or Postnatal Anxiety (PNA), the reason I haven't delved too far into these subjects yet is simple. If you are suffering to the point you fear the blues have engulfed

---

*PANDA via Deloitte Access Economics. The cost of perinatal depression in Australia. Report. Post and Antenatal Depression Association 2012

you, you're going to need more than a chapter in a book. This is a conversation that needs to fall on the ears of a professional & before that your partner or a loved one. And soon. Very soon (...as in now).

If you are not coping, if you feel erratic, unable to hold focus, foggy, lethargic, or fatigued. If you have extreme fears or patches of deep sadness or panic. If you feel teary, out of control, on edge, or unsafe. If you don't trust your thoughts, your actions. If you don't recognise yourself or your loved ones. If you feel confused, angry, completely useless and as if you're not good enough.

If you feel like you're drowning & you don't want to hold your baby, or even be near your baby please know two things;

1. You Are Not Alone and;
2. There Are Brilliant People Just Waiting To Help You

Let people in, even when you feel you'd rather be alone. Tell them you're not coping & that you need help. This isn't a failure, this is brave and to be applauded. Well done Mumma.

I'd also urge you to check out PANDA (www.panda.org.au and @pandanational). As noted on their website, "PANDA (Perinatal Anxiety & Depression Australia) supports women, men, and families across Australia affected by anxiety and depression during pregnancy and in the first year of parenthood. PANDA operates Australia's only National Helpline for individuals and their families to recover from perinatal anxiety and depression, a serious illness that affects up to one in five expecting or new Mums and one in ten expecting or new Dads."

For a real-life story or something that may offer you a way to relate, there is a wonderful podcast by **Beyond The Bump,** that explores one of the co-host's battle with PND after the birth of her third child. Her uncontrollable state spiraled to the point she asked to be driven to the emergency room as even the sight of her own three children had become unrecognisable. They looked different to her and she was fearful and unable to explain what was happening to her. The episode is called "Jayde - Journey With PND and PNA After Her Third Baby." It's a fantastic listen.

You'll be ok, just focus on being very emphatic with your state of mind. You're in a pitch-black, cold & unidentifiable room. You need someone to guide you to the light switch before you can find the way out. There are people within your community who can do this with you but they need to know you're trapped first. So that flare in your hand? You know it's there …. fire it. Ask for help.

EXERCISE

Pre Baby Body … a phrase we should all delete from our minds as we are not our Pre Baby Self anymore. We are our Post Baby Self. Our Post Baby Self is super lovely if you spend the time & get to know her. She's kind, fun, giving & generous.

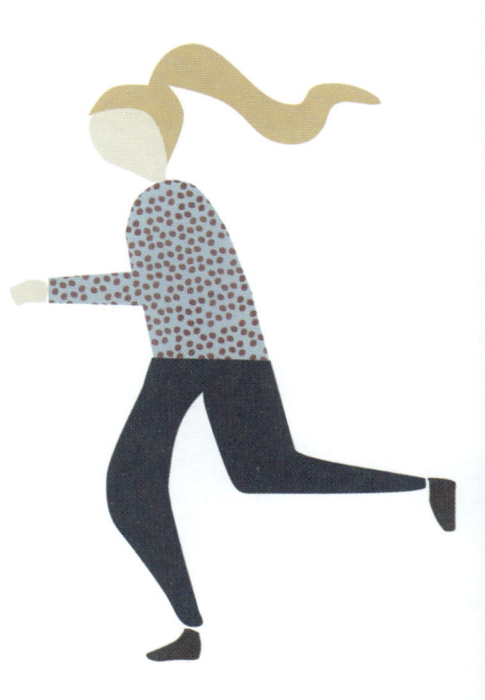

But she is also very tired. She is acutely aware that her skinny jeans don't button up at the moment, she knows she looks daggy in her maternity bra and she can feel that her belly is soft & see that her eyes are dark. There is no need to remind your Post Baby Self that her boobs look like something off Embarrassing Bodies. She's postpartum, she ain't blind. And her top that's on backward and inside out? I can assure you, she knows. She is ok with it. See what I mean? Your Post Baby Self is a legend. She just goes with the flow.

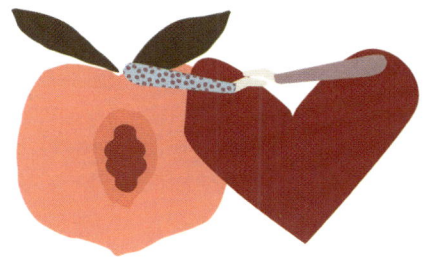

She is doing her best to stay awake and not cry. She is trying hard not to wet herself and she's remembering to politely nod at the two million pieces of advice that fly her way each day by the hundreds of visitors ... who she is truly appreciative of as they always seem to bring banana bread & quiche. She loves banana bread and quiche.

So please give this lovely las a break.

The postpartum period is not the time to sign yourself up for a bootcamp. It's the time to rest, nurse, heal & pay close attention to your body. Not just your belly & your thighs, but your pelvic floor, your abdomen, your internal organs, your back, your muscles, ligaments & tissues.

The subject of exercise is another subject this book doesn't delve into too deeply as returning to exercise is something that requires personalised guidance & feedback. Your pregnancy, your birth & your recovery will be miles apart from any other woman. We are all unique in terms of the condition of our bodies during the weeks and months that follow birth, so I'd say it's imperative to chat with a professional before returning to a workout.

You might be busting to get a sweat going in a yoga class, a spin class, or simply a light jog. You might think it's safe to do a few squats while you rock your baby to sleep or clock up some sit-ups when you're on the floor doing tummy time.

Whatever you crave doing, get the tick of approval from your women's health physio, your maternal health nurse, or your GP beforehand. Be patient as you never know what kind of extra damage you could cause.

On the topic of exercise & the body, the postpartum period is also probably not the right time to dabble in Paleo or FODMAP or get lost in the latest fad diet. Now is the time to nourish your belly in goodness … delicious goodness! Fresh fruits, vegetables, wholemeal bread, rice & grains. Meat, eggs, nuts, fish, dairy, and plenty of omegas 3's. And water. Gulp up so much water! A good meal, rest and just enjoying your precious new baby is all you need to focus on right now. Let your body chill out & heal. It'll thank you in the long run!

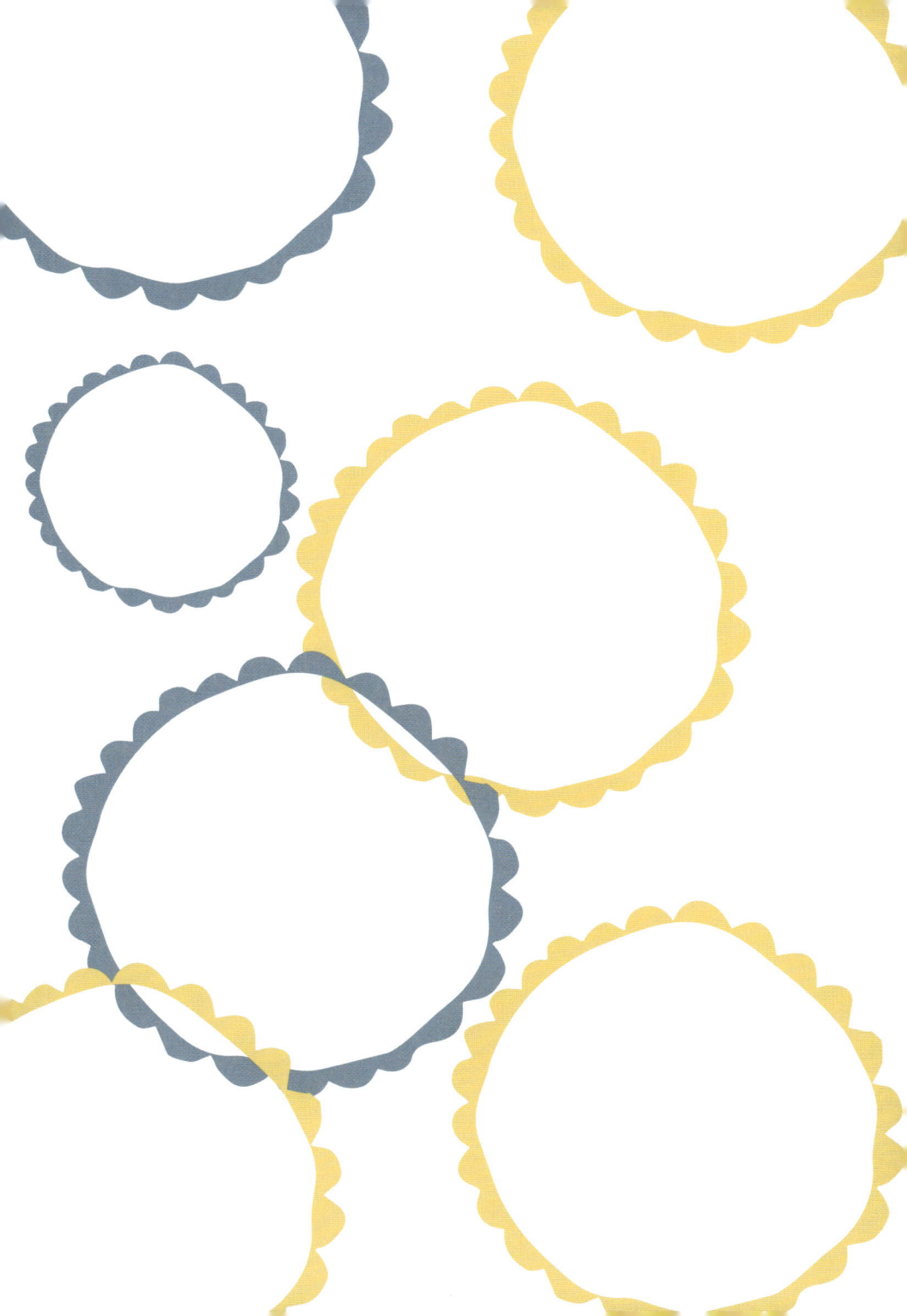

quick hack

LACTATIN' BAKIN'

If you feel as though your milk is drying out a little, the first thing to do is to have a chat with a lactation consultant, your midwife or your GP. Whilst you wait for an appointment, however, remember to drink lots of water & load up on healthy snacks such as oats & dates. Or, if you want to get busy in the kitchen, why not bake some boobie bikkies!

There are so many fabulous recipes on the world wide web that cater for all preferences, allergies & food intolerances. For now, I can almost guarantee that all of the recipes you find will require the following list of ingredients. So when you next pop out to the store, add these to your list!

SHOPPING LIST

- ◊ Oats
- ◊ Brewers yeast
- ◊ Self-raising wholemeal flour (or normal flour + baking soda)
- ◊ Coconut oil or butter
- ◊ Coconut sugar or brown sugar ... or you can use dates or currents for sweetness
- ◊ Eggs
- ◊ Flaxseed meal
- ◊ Salt
- ◊ For taste: Vanilla extract, cranberries, chocolate chips (dark or milk), vanilla, cinnamon, coconut ... the world is your boobie cookie.

If you're not the baking type, you can buy ready-made lactation cookies online or at larger chemists such as Chemist Warehouse. Just keep in mind, the sugar content is likely to be much higher when it comes to pre-prepared goodies.

Food For Thought: My bestfriend made me a batch of homemade boobie bikkies when my bub was about 2 or 3 months old. They were delicious and so effective! I froze the batch & munched on one per night, alongside a few fresh dates.

So if you are heading to a baby shower soon, a nice gift idea might be to bake the expecting Mumma a batch of biks for her freezer. It was quite honestly one of the best gifts I received. My baby, my boobs and my belly were one happy trio.

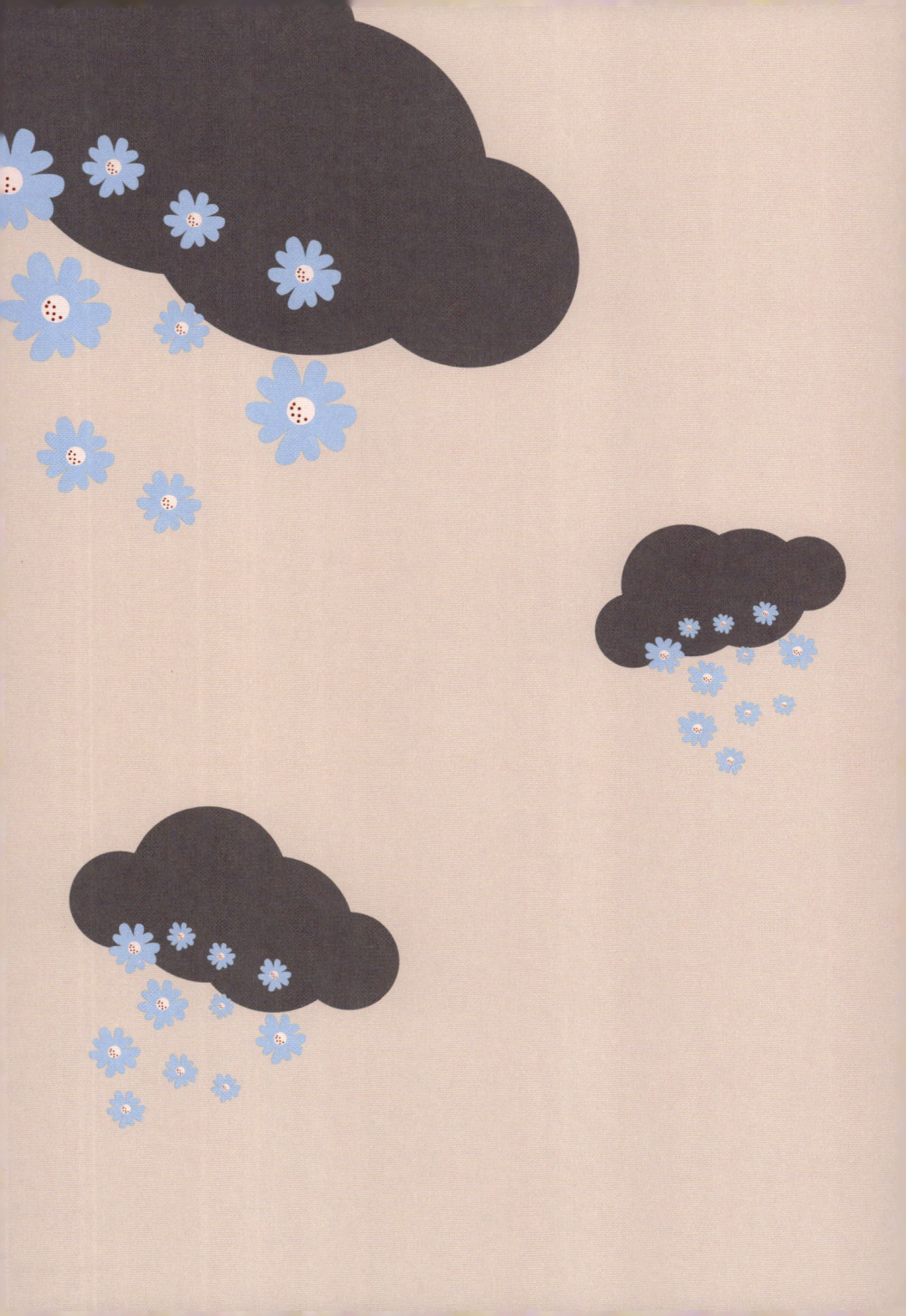

CHAPTER 11

When It's Not Postnatal Depression

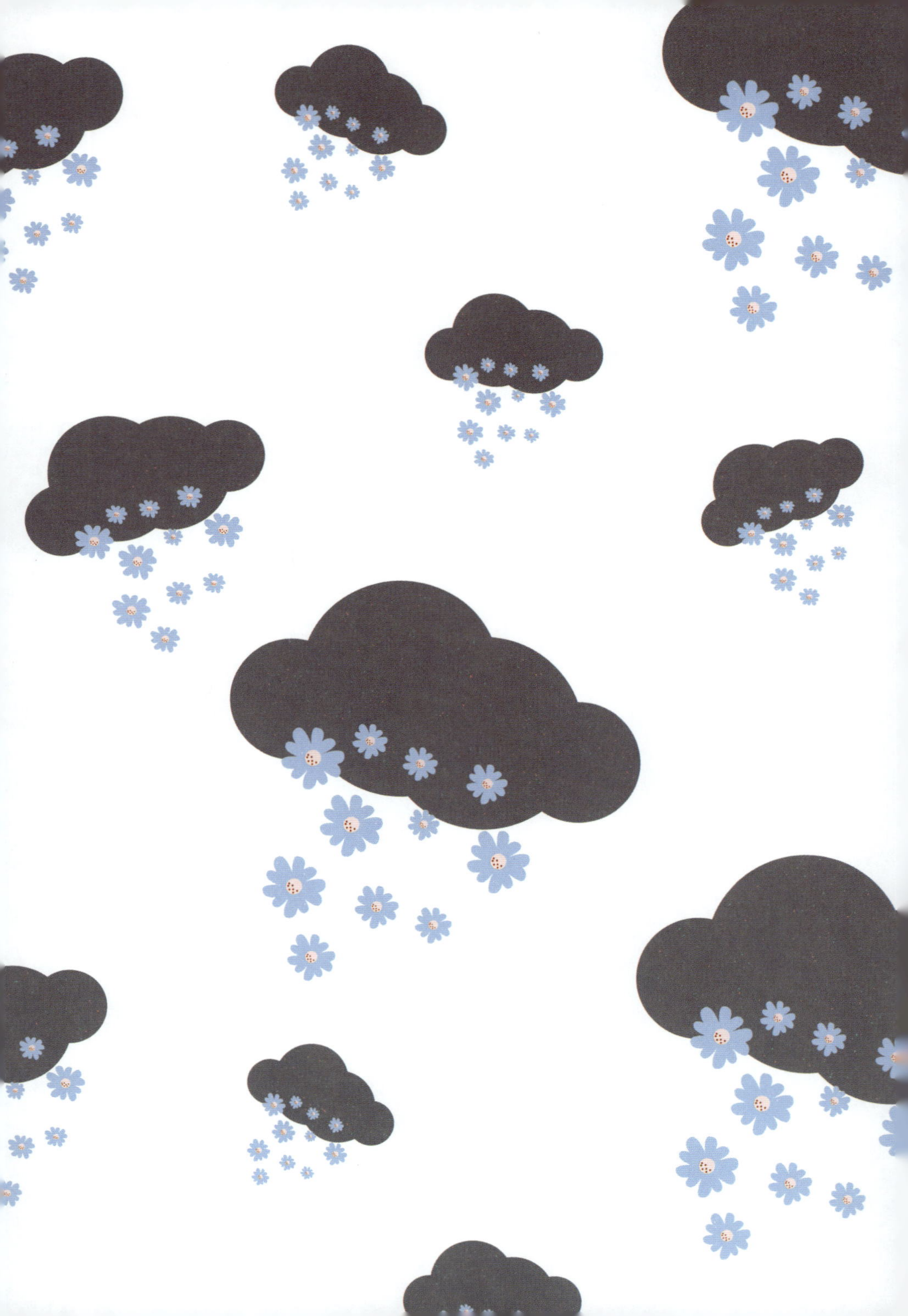

Let's take the postnatal out of postnatal depression for a moment and just focus on mothers who have suffered from a mental health issue prior to becoming pregnant or having their baby. Whether it's depression you've previously tangoed with or anxiety or anything else - the introduction of a baby in your life shouldn't encourage you to ignore the illness. Yes, you are a mother now. But you are still you. While postpartum life brings change, some things in your life will stay the same … like my heinous ability to share food. I assumed motherhood would make me so generously giving. As it turns out, not if it's fruit toast.

While I will be very careful not to generalise this subject as it is so varied and unique to each individual, I'll inject a little of myself into the text as I myself have danced with depression in the past. So for those like me, hopefully you'll find an inch of comfort here.

For years I've lived with what's commonly known as a text book chemical imbalance. When I'm in the thick of it & my centre is frowning to one side, I feel disconnected from what is familiar to me and to my life. Friday night loses its buzz. Sunday morning loses its ease. Everything melts into a flat puddle & I become a spectator of my own life. I can see the dinner party where my family & friends sit … I just can't get to the table because there is a big glass wall in front of me. The glass is heavy & it is fogged. Put simply, during my patches of grey, I'm unable to firmly ground my feet, leaving me floating around like an aloof, detached bubble.

When I was 22 & living away from home, I took myself to the GP as my bubble had started to stray a little too far from home. I was nervous for the first time. From that day onwards I was properly diagnosed and I started to take medication.

Along with exercise, a good diet and an eye out for my triggers (when you've known this feeling for some time, you come to know your tiggers very well), my life changed for the better. The glass wall vanished & the bubble landed safely on the ground.

Since then, I've come off the medication a few times - I can't explain it but on a few occasions I've simply felt an urge to go solo. Periods without it can last months or even a year, but when I see or feel a trigger, I go back to the path I know will lead me home. Life is too short to be lost when you know exactly where you need to me.

When I fell pregnant, I had a discussion with my GP about whether or not I'd stay on the meds throughout the 9 months. Many pregnant women do stay on their medication - I must stress that point. I however decided to come off them and see how I went. If at any point I felt that the bubble was whisking me away, I knew what to do.

Luckily for me I got through the 9 month pregnancy with no issue. I adored pregnancy and the devilish little D-man kept his sweet distance. 6 months into motherhood the continuation of my ability to get up everyday and feel good, positive and like myself continued. I was over the moon, a little surprised if I am to be honest, and so insanely grateful.

Just after the 6 month mark, I can't remember the exact moment, or even if there was an exact moment, but I started to float. For some reason I never thought twice about whether or not it could have been postnatal depression … it just felt too damn familiar to be anything else but what I knew. I made an appointment with the GP, had a long chat, asked a zillion questions (what if, what if, what if…), and returned to my usual dose.

Do I feel disappointed? Or ashamed? Or as if I've failed?

NO WAY! I feel bloody lucky that I have the option to feel good. I feel grateful that, unlike so many other people, I know my triggers and I know my cure. I feel indebted to our wonderful healthcare system & just so overjoyed that I can wake up everyday knowing I can give my son, my whole family, all of me. Every inch.

If you have dealt with mental health hiccups in the past … then you know. It is a sure way to an isolated loneliness that no-one should ever have to endure if there is an option to escape it.

Pregnancy & breastfeeding do create many hurdles and ignite serious discussions about risks & potential side effects. This bit cannot be disregarded nor can it be sugarcoated. Having said that, a possible cure shouldn't be cast to the side due to fear or assumption. Please speak to a medical healthcare professional openly, candidly and promptly if you feel as if you need help. Access to help is a life luxury.

I will always say your baby needs to be the priority in your life when you are a parent. Of course. I will also say that as your priority, your wellbeing is paramount. They need you to be well. Just remember, looking after yourself is looking after your baby.

THANK YOU

Thank you

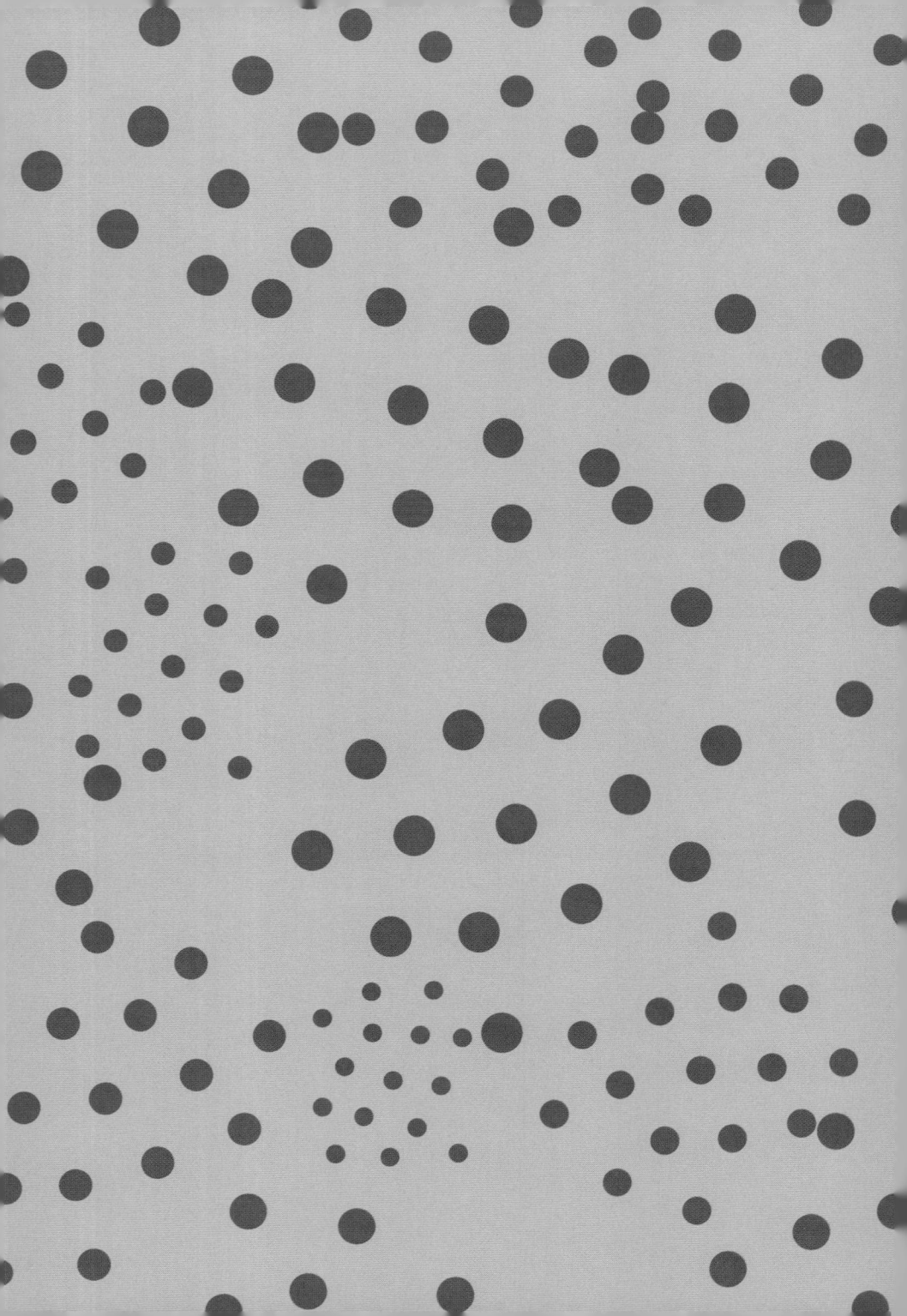

Thank you to everyone for reading along. I hope that AFTERWARDS has provided and will continue to provide a light and safe space for you to hide away when you crave a little solace & support. Just remember, from one Mum to another, having a baby is as wonderful as it is tough. And I've only had ONE baby … and for just ONE year. Despite my experiences not being as ripe or as aged as that glass of red we all dream of … at 11am … over the last 13months with my son, I've learned more than I have in my lifetime. The biggest lesson? There is never just the one solution to a problem. There is an ocean of ways to cope and survive. Celebrating others and holding back every ounce of judgment needs to be in the rulebook of Mums everywhere.

Be kind. To yourself … and to everyone around you.

I'm sure the adventure of motherhood will continue to throw all of us into days where we feel that we have only enough energy to exist in a dazed & confused fog … but with every moment of "WTF?", another moment of pure, surreal, indescribable and magnificent wonder will follow. Those are the moments worth hanging in for.

Thank you to the uber fabulous & spectacularly talented Catherine Malady for all of her superb illustrations. Catherine is one of the most naturally gifted people I know. Her work is charming, sweet and always so delightfully warm. Catherine is a "Watch This Space," kinda gal … with a portfolio to date that is filled with utter brilliance, she has oodles of magic yet to be seen by the world, so keep your eye on the name Catherine Malady (you can start by following her new Instagram account @my_cat_is_a_hat). CTG, you're wonderful, marvellous & very much adored. I appreciate your time on this book so much, and I appreciate YOU for simply being YOU.

When it comes to the physical & human biology related side of things … the Pelvic Floor & the female anatomy at large, my longtime & highly qualified friend Phoebe Marinovich, has generously contributed guidance, consult and highly valuable advice into these pages. Phoebe has edited my words along the way to ensure that my "fluffiness" is legitimate, correct and safe. I urge all women to follow along @f_e_m_m_e___silasphysio, and watch for Phoebe's regular delivery of tips and advice. A warm, giving and highly empathetic individual, Phoebe should be a part of every woman's pregnancy & postpartum experience. This book would be nothing without you, so thank you darling Phoebs x

For all matters on beauty & skin … Natalie Beaumont & Tiffany Smith-Shiels are the brilliant gals to credit here! Two of the most adored beauty therapists, both Nat & Tiff go far beyond their fields of expertise to constantly ensure the advice they offer is highly personalised and well researched. They have the gift of making their clientele feel comfortable, beautiful and safe … and on top of that, they have smiles & souls worthy of gold.

Sophie Outhwaite … Mumma of two and midwife to so many lucky women. Soph you're a superwomen! Thank you so much for your words of wisdom & for sharing your experiences and advice with not only myself, but with the readers of this book. I value your time immensely and hope that everyone follows Soph at @minimalistmidwife for everything they need to know about Mumma-life. Soph is the most relaxed, rational & realistic woman on this topic. A true gem.

Sarah Mitchell who shared her wisdom and knowledge about all things boobs! Sarah is a treat. A sweet delight. A talented & caring person with a knowledge of wealth in her field. I am enormously grateful to you Sar, thank you! I bet many women will find comfort and guidance within your words.

Chantelle Otten, our resident sexologist. I am so fortunate to have had the chance to include Chantelle's words of wisdom in the book and I must thank my adored friend Georgie Saggers for the kind introduction. Chantelle, @chantelle_otten_sexologist, is a woman in high demand around the country as let's face it, she is wildly incredible! With so much recent candidness regarding the global conversation around female liberation, Chantelle is an authentic voice that captures the attention of so many. A luxuriant & kind hearted supporter of all women & their road to true pleasure ... Chantelle you're precious. Thank you!

Liz Manning, my cousin! I couldn't be more grateful for your time and energy editing this book! Another working Mumma of two little cutie-patooties, another modern day superwoman! Spelling, grammar and creating sentences that follow the guidelines of legitimate English has never been my forte. Liz's sharp skills are beyond! For correcting the following sentence in particular, "... after delivering your big bugga" ... to "...delivering your big bubba", it is safe to say, you've saved the essence of this book. Cheers to you!

Stacie Lucas from GOYA Studio! The most amazing designer (and Mum!), with an eye for clean, fresh creations. Thank you for working with me to design a book that feels calm, friendly and inviting. For new Mums who are tired & overwhelmed by the millions of things going through their mind at any one time, having a safe space to melt into makes a huge difference to the day. I couldn't be more grateful to have you on board.

To my own MUM and my own SON! I love that you two are the soul reason this book exists. Mum, for getting me through the newborn, toddler, primary school, teenage, early adult and now this new "motherhood" stage of my life ... I really do think you have super powers. To the moon & back, I cherish you more.

Hamish my baby boy ... thank you for providing me with laughs, cuddles and oodles of joy. You are my little fella, my little man, my little love. If and when my mothering skills are a tad underwhelming, I promise you this ... I will never stop trying to be the home you crave racing back to. I know one day you'll build your own life, but your Mumma's front door will never be closed to you. You are out of this world kiddo. Thank goodness you're here.

To Willy. My husband & my best mate. Thank you for being my co-pilot during this parenthood adventure. While we have no real clue what we're doing most days, it's safe to say we're having the absolute time of our lives raising our Hamish. Our chaos is our bliss, our son is our sanctuary. You're a wonderful Dadda. You're a spectacular person. You're the reason I'm lucky enough to be a Mum … and you are the best goddam swaddle-er to ever walk this earth. Mothers around the world salute you.

And to all the people who have helped my motherhood story … friends, family, midwives, GP's, Postcast'ers, bloggers, Instagram'ers and the very patient people at the chemist who must think to themselves, "What the hell does she need now!?!" … thank you.

I'm sure I'll re-read this book when I have future babies and I'll think to myself … "I was so naive to think that one baby, after one year was tough!" But to my future self re-reading this & thinking that exact thought … put a cork in it lady. It's all relative.

Ciao for now

xox

If you got to the end of the book, thank you again for reading! I'd love to hear from you at tori@jandvco.com

The AFTERWARDS chronicles aims to continue & expand, so if you have any thoughts, feelings or emotions bubbling away on the topic of motherhood, let me know!

Enjoy a wonderful day!

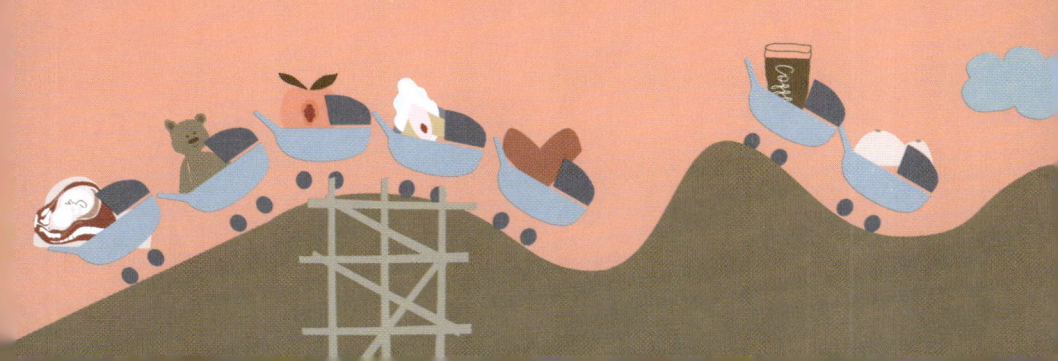

You are my sunshine, my only sunshine
You make me happy when skies are gray
You'll never know dear, how much I love you
Please don't take my sunshine away

                              JOHNNY CASH

YOUR OWN NOTES, THOUGHTS & FEELINGS....

Pass it on to a friend, sibling or maybe even your baby in time, keep the notes for next time or simply save & cherish the memory.

....

....

....

....

....

....

....

....

....

....

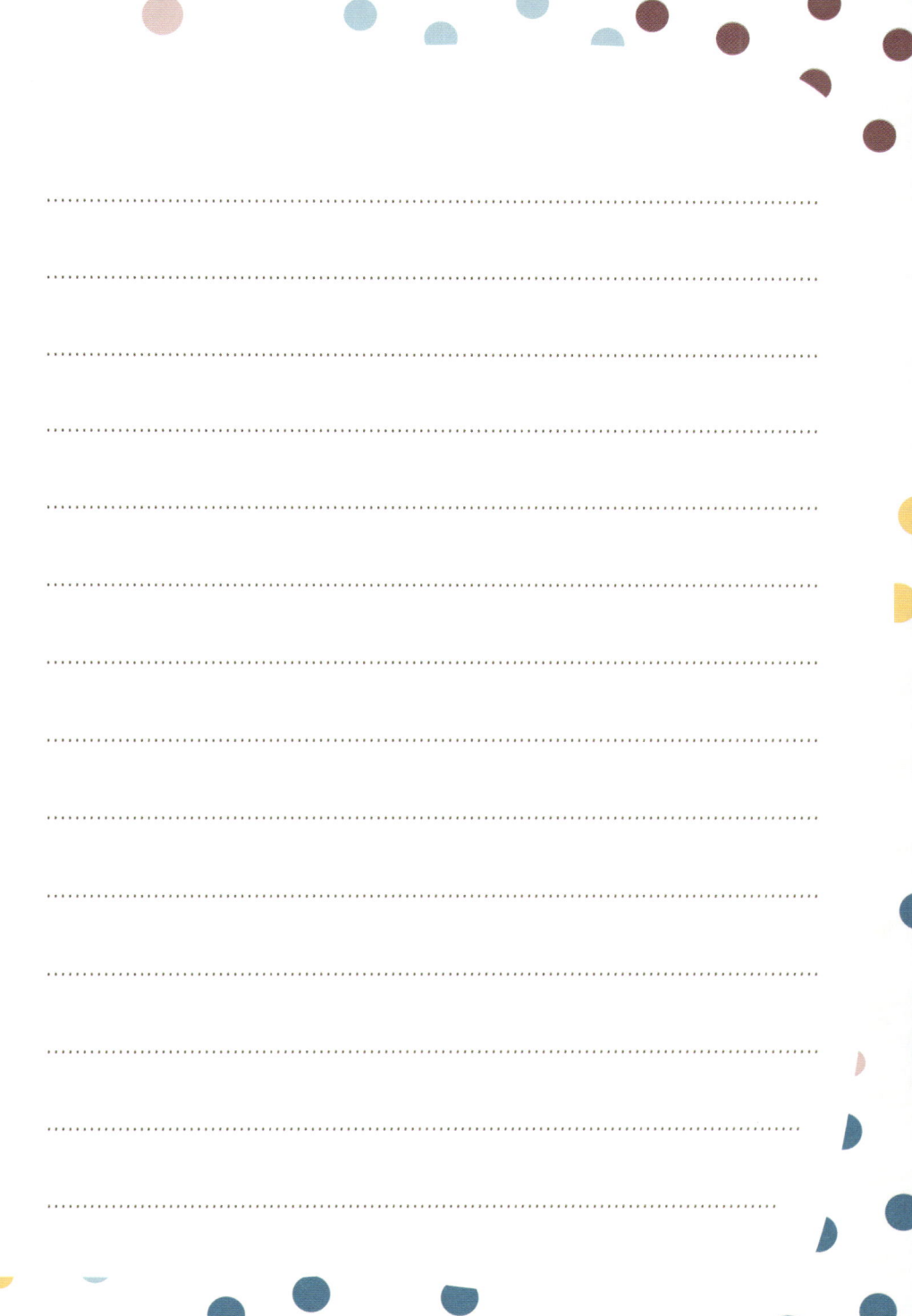

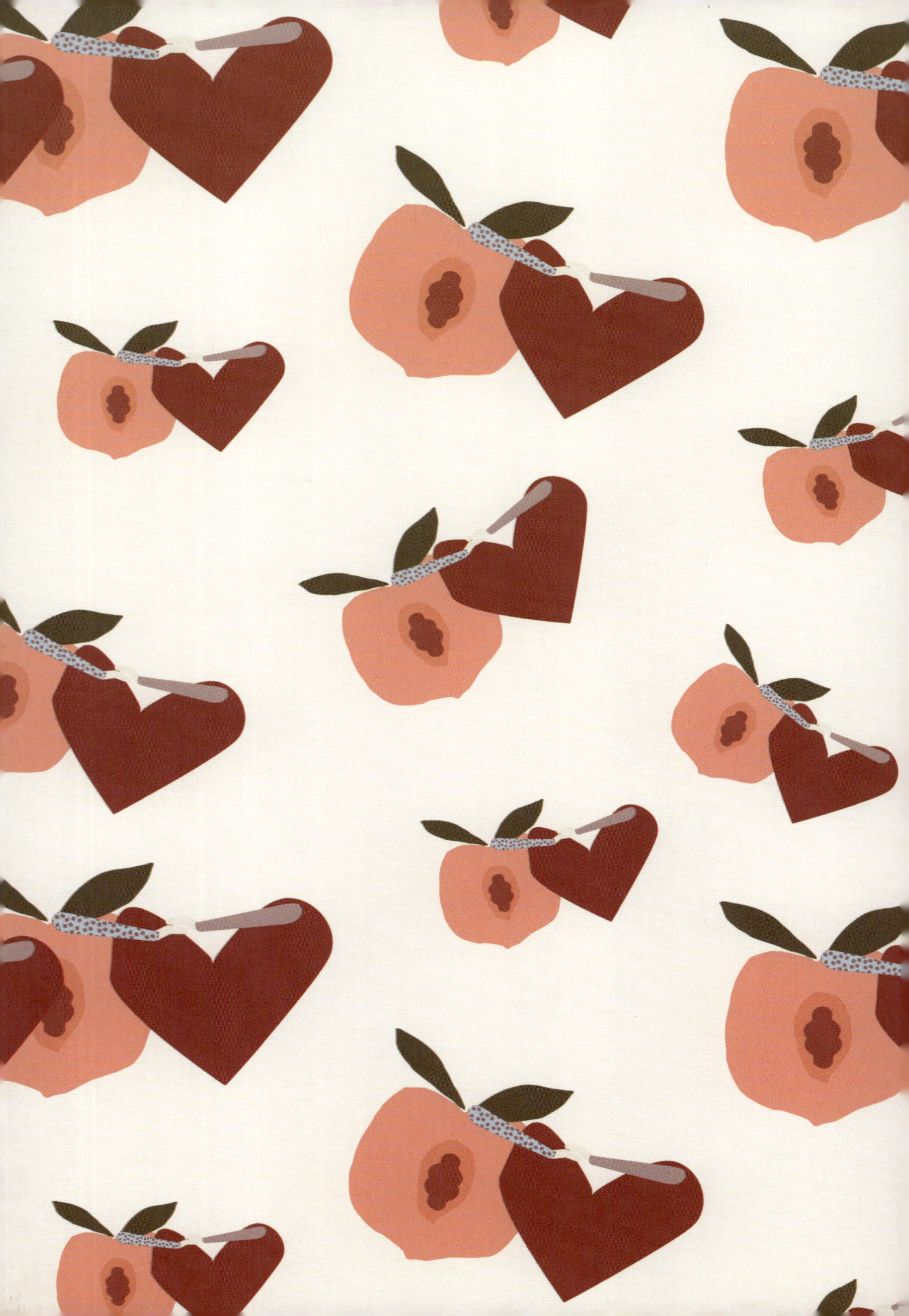